U0093941

Taiwan Can Help

For All The World To See

讓世界看見臺灣

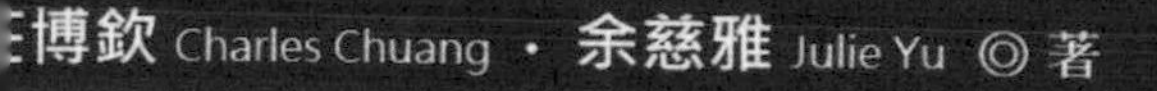

莊博欽 Charles Chuang ・ 余慈雅 Julie Yu ◎著

前言 Origin

溫暖慈悲的粉紅台灣

A heartwarming and compassionate pink Taiwan

新冠肺炎的疫情漫延全世界

許多議題不停的在紛飛

As the pandemic of COVID-19 rampaged the world, many issues have aroused in the air.

WHO can help?（註：1）

太過衝突！

不想只是登在紐約時報自嗨個一天就沒了～

我用實際出版發行 Taiwan can help 上架亞馬遜，讓全世界永遠可以真正看見台灣！

在世界衛生與全球健康問題緊張的環境之下 Taiwan can help.

不宜用嚴肅的政治問題再去衝撞升高緊張，逼迫世界選邊站……成為 Troublemaker.

WHO can help? (note:1)

There has been too much conflict!

I don't want to post on the New York Times for one day only for a limited number of people to see and be gone on the next~

Under the tense circumstances where the WHO and global health are facing tough challenges, Taiwan can help.

Therefore, I'm taking actions by publishing Taiwan can Help on Amazon for the whole world to see Taiwan truly!

It is inappropriate using political issues to heighten the tension, forcing the world to pick a side, and at the same time, inadvertently, make us seem like a troublemaker.

事實上，台灣還有「粉紅口罩」（註：2）的溫馨議題、台灣還有白沙屯媽祖的「粉紅超跑」（註：3）放送慈悲……台灣還有許多美食、旅遊、文化、科技與藝術人文等多元的議題值得讓全世界看到。

As a matter of fact, in Taiwan, there are heart-warming topics such as "Pink mask" (note:2), and "Pink Supercar" of Mazu in

Baishatun that delivers compassion, not to mention the many diverse topics about food, travel, culture, technology, arts that are worth the world to see.

當前全球的疫情 Taiwan can help. 我們擁有真正的美好實力，就讓粉紅台灣療癒全世界！

Taiwan can help with the current pandemic situation in the globe, and we have the ability to do so, so let pink Taiwan heal the world!

這本書以中、英文對照印行，台灣及亞馬遜同步於全世界發行，這也代表是一種台灣與全世界的溝通意義，特別是繁體中文才是正統華文的傳承，全世界想要學習華文的人可以藉由這本書來認識真正美麗的中文，台灣人也可以藉由這本書來學英文，在文字交流之中，同時學習與傳遞的是正統中華文化的傳承在台灣。

This book is published in both Chinese and English, simultaneously in Taiwan and Amazon, and distributed to all over the world, also signifying the communication between Taiwan and the whole world. What's more, traditional Chinese is the inheritance of orthodox Chinese. Anyone in the world who desires to learn Chinese can learn the true beauty of Chinese through this book. Taiwanese people can also learn English through this book. In the exchange of words and literature, what we learn and transmit is the heritage of orthodox Chinese culture in Taiwan.

發行人 / 范世華

Publisher / Fan Shi-Hua

註 1：新冠肺炎疫情爆發之初，台灣曾警告 WHO (世界衛生組織) 因應漫延的防疫措施，卻因為政治因素而被漠視，並引發 WHO 秘書長譚德塞與台灣一連串互嗆的口水戰。而後台灣網紅 Youtuber 發起募資刊登「WHO can help?」的廣告於紐約時報，用以諷刺 WHO (世界衛生組織) 不中立，有失維護世界衛生防疫之責。

Note 1: In the early days of COVID-19 outbreak, Taiwan has warned the WHO (World Health Organization) that prevention measures should be taken, but the message was ignored due to political issues, subsequently triggered a series of heated exchanges between WHO Chief Tedros Adhanom Ghebreyesus and Taiwan. Later, Taiwanese influencer Youtuber initiated a fundraiser and published an ad "WHO can help?" in the New York Times to satirize the WHO (World Health Organization)'s non-neutrality and failure to maintain the responsibility of safeguarding world health and pandemic prevention.

註 2：台灣在防疫過程中，疾管署防疫專線接獲民眾投訴，說有一名小學男童因為分配到粉紅色口罩，擔心遭同學議論而不想去上學。結果，隔天部長和官員們就真的戴上粉紅色口罩登場記者會，也讓配帶粉紅口罩成為富有溫暖故事的一股風潮。

Note 2: During the epidemic prevention process in Taiwan, the Disease Control Department’s Epidemic Prevention Hotline received complaints from the public that a primary schoolboy was assigned a pink mask and did not want to go to school for fear of being talked about by classmates. As a result, the ministers and officials wore pink masks for the press conference the next day, making wearing pink masks a trend.

註 3：敬拜媽祖是台灣傳統的一個民間信仰，每年都會舉行一次媽祖進香儀式，信眾跟隨媽祖繞境之活動盛大有如嘉年華會，其中白沙屯媽祖鑾轎轎頂因覆蓋一層粉紅色帆布，用於遮雨、保護、點綴鑾轎，柔合的粉紅色也突顯代表著媽祖的慈悲心，而祂行進的路線除了讓人難以預測之外，其步程速度有時飛快，因此被信眾形容為「粉紅超跑」。
Note 3: Mazu worshipping is a traditional folk belief in Taiwan. An incense ceremony for Mazu is held every year. The activities of believers to follow Mazu around the territory are as grand as a carnival. Among them, the Baishatun Mazu Luang sedan chair is covered with a pink canvas to shelter it from the rain, protect and embellish the Luang sedan chair. The soft pink color also highlights the compassion of Mazu. Moreover, the route of its path is unpredictable, and the walking speed is incredibly fast, described by believers as "Pink Supercar."

序 Preface

臺灣是個遠比大家想像中還要適合居住與發展的地方。

Taiwan is a place far more suitable for living and development than people think.

2020 年 1 月 21 號，臺灣首例新冠肺炎確診。

January 21, 2020, the first case of novel coronavirus infection in Taiwan confirmed

在疫情爆發的初期，我對疫情的想法並不樂觀，因為在疫情開始的期間，正好是我重拾過去，展開我創業旅途的時候。只是時不運我，我開始與其他企業主一同面臨因疫情影響的經濟危機與業務緊縮的問題。

When the pandemic first broke out, I was not optimistic about it at all. I had just started picking up my life, about to embark on entrepreneurship. But time was not on my side, like other business owners, I started facing the economic crisis and business austerity under the pandemic’s influence.

我在 2019 年 12 月我開始了我創業一連串的規劃，我的規劃是提供一個可以服務中小企業創業者，讓他們能透過我的服務建立品牌、加速成長的網站平台，我的經營宗旨是讓中小企業主無論是想要品牌設計、募資企劃、網站架設、搜尋引擎優化還是出版行銷，都能透過我的網站有效地被滿足需求並得到期望的報酬率，有效獲得企業的加速成長。
On December 12, 2019, I started a series of planning for starting my own business. The plan is to provide an online platform to assist small and medium business owners in establishing their brands through my services, including brand design, fundraising plans, website setup, SEO (search engine optimization), publishing, and marketing, which can all be found through my website. The mission statement is to provide integrated services to effectively satisfy all businesses' needs to help their growth and reach expected returns.

只是，這次的疫情不光影響到一般民眾的情緒，更讓企業主對今後的市場發展產生了恐懼（疫情期間各國各標的股價不約而同地呈現下滑的趨勢，同時業務緊縮使得愈來愈多企業關門大吉），這個疫情的蝴蝶效應也導致了我的網站無法有效地將我的服務傳達給企業主，就算是看到了我服務的企業主也會因為害怕這次疫情會讓他們損失更多金錢而不願意或躊躇不前，這個惡性循環使人絕望，也讓我產生想要放棄的想法。

However, this pandemic not only affected the emotions of the general public, but it also inflicted panic on business owners about the prospects of the future market (as reflected by the drastic drop in the stock market in different countries, and the sharp fall in business which also leads to more and more companies to shut down). The pandemic's butterfly effect also led to my website's inability to communicate my services to business owners effectively. Even the bus e money.iness owners who saw my services would be reluctant or hesitant because they were afraid that the pandemic would cost them mor This vicious circle made people despair and made me want to give up.

2020 年 4 月 14 日，當日臺灣無新增確診個案。

April 14, 2020, no additional cases of coronavirus disease were found.

直到臺灣發布第一次的零確診消息，我看到了臺灣經濟復甦的理由，也燃起了一道希望的曙光。

When Taiwan announced news of the first no additional new case of infection for the day, I saw reasons for the economic recovery in Taiwan and a spark of hope.

這段消息後續帶來的連鎖反應不僅讓我機會重拾信心，更讓我有希望繼續開始我的創業旅途，儘管在這段期間有部分民眾因為零確診的消息變得更加警惕與恐懼，但這並不影響大多數臺灣人產生了戰勝疫情的希望，同時這也讓臺灣人更有自信地堅持抗疫,並為這個世界多付出一份心力。

The chain effects brought by the news not only made me picked up faith but also endowed me with the hope of continuing my entrepreneurial journey. Despite some people becoming more alert and fearful due to the news of zero diagnosis, it does not affect the belief of most Taiwanese people, that the disease will be defeated, given them the confidence in continuing the campaign, and making more efforts for the world.

因為大家的努力，臺灣正在逐漸康復。

Due to everyone's effort, Taiwan is gradually recovering.

現在，臺灣可以幫助其他人了！

Now, Taiwan can help others!

而我也決定，將臺灣這片土地帶給我的希望回饋給其他世界各地的民眾。有了臺灣，讓我能在疫情期間安穩度日，有了臺灣，讓我因疫情變得渺茫的創業旅途再次有了希望。於是我寫了這本書，我希望能因我的文字，讓看到這本書的各國人民能因為臺灣的成功重拾希望，臺灣做到了！你們當然也可以。

Due to everyone's effort, Taiwan is gradually recovering. And I also decided to give back to people worldwide the hope that this land of Taiwan has brought to me. With Taiwan, I can live in peace during the pandemic. With Taiwan, I have faith again for my once seemingly perilous entrepreneurial journey. So I wrote this book, hoping that through my words, people of all countries who read this book can regain hope due to Taiwan's success, Taiwan did it! You can do it too!

"讓世界重新燃起希望的燈火，讓世界一同戰勝瘟疫的恐懼。"

Let the world rekindle the light of hope, let the world overcome the fear of plague together

煋蜂品牌加速坊 Charles Chuang

MarsBee ProjectSquare Charles Chuang

目錄

前言 溫暖慈悲的粉紅台灣 5
序 11

第一章 臺灣零確診
I. 昔日大敵－曾經我們有一個叫做 SARS 的敵人 25
II. 孤島求生－在四處環海的孤島上我們只能生存 37
III. 反射神經－過去的慘烈戰疫烙印在人們的心中 49
IV. 防毒面具－想要隔絕毒氣你需要一張防毒面具 59
V. 超前部署－事前的規劃永遠都是最安全的選項 73

第二章 臺灣是什麼
I. 地球之島－這個地方有著全世界的氣候與美景 91
II. 美食天堂－這個地方有著各國各地的美食選擇 103
III. 傳送之門－這個地方擁有非常方便快速的交通 121
IV. 炎黃古跡－這個地方保存著昔日的文明與禮儀 131

Table of Content

Origin A heartwarming and compassionate pink Taiwan 5

Preface 11

Chapter 1 Zero Confirmed cases in Taiwan

I. Past Enemy-Once upon a time, we had an enemy called SARS 25

II. Survival on the Island of Isolation- On an island surrounded by sea, we could only survive on our own 37

III. Reflective Nerves-The bitter memories of past combat against disease are branded in people's heart 49

IV. Gas Mask- To block out poisonous gas, you need a gas mask 59

V. Advance Preparations-Early planning is always the safest choice 73

Chapter 2 What is Taiwan

I. An Island on earth-This place has the best climate and views in the world 91

II. Food Paradise-This place provides culinary options from all over the world 103

III. Portal-This place has very convenient and rapid transportation 121

IV. Chinese Cultural Heritage-This place preserves past culture and etiquette 131

第三章　臺灣能助你
I. 資源助你－或許你們需要更多的資源隔絕病毒 145
II. 技術助你－或許你們需要更多的技術制止病毒 155

第四章　戰疫知識共享
I. 戰術背包－如果你要出門，你得要帶這些東西 167
II. 防疫功夫－如果你想防疫，你得要會這些招式 175

後記 180

Chapter 3 Taiwan Can Help

I. In Resources-Perhaps you need more resources to block the virus 145

II. In technology-Perhaps you need more technology support in stopping the virus 155

Chapter 4 Share Knowledge in fighting the pandemic

I. Tactical Backpack-If you are going out, you should pack these 167

II. Disease Prevention Measures- If you want to keep away from the virus, you should know these. 175

Epilogue 180

護臺灣、助世界

臺灣能幫忙，而且臺灣正在幫忙

Taiwan can help
and Taiwan is helping

第一章
Chapter 1

臺灣零確診
Zero confirmed cases in Taiwan

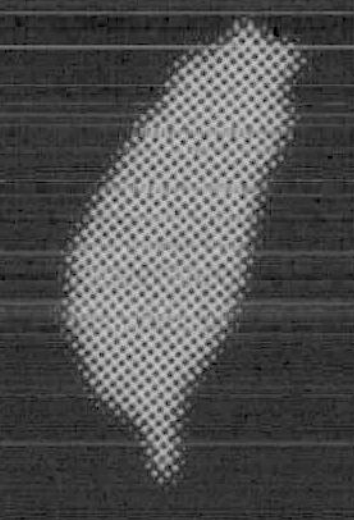

昔日大敵

Past Enemy

曾經我們有一個叫做 SARS 的敵人

Once upon a time, we had an enemy called SARS

2020 年 4 月 14 日，當日臺灣無新增確診個案，並於 4 月 26 日至 5 月 1 日期間連續保持零確診紀錄。

On April 14, 2020, Taiwan reported no new confirmed cases and kept the record of zero confirmed cases from April 26 to May 1.

臺灣是一個防疫措施做得非常優秀的國家，除了得天獨厚的地理環境及政治生態外，我們之所以能防疫的如此迅速，並獲得防疫成功，這或許要歸功於我們過去的敵人－**SARS**。

Taiwan is a country with outstanding performance in pandemic prevention measures. Apart from its one of a kind geographical environment and political ecology,

We have been able to contain the pandemic so quickly and successfully may be attributed to our past enemy, **SARS**.

SARS，全稱為嚴重急性呼吸道症候群（Severe Acute Respiratory Syndrome），最早出現於 2002 年秋冬之際在中國大陸廣東省一帶，是由未知病原體引發的非典型肺炎，在 2003 年 2 月擴散至臺灣等東南亞地區，於 3 月底世界衛生組織向全球發出警訊，並將此種疾病正式命名為 SARS。

Severe Acute Respiratory Syndrome, also known as **SARS**, atypical pneumonia caused by unknown pathogens, first appeared in the area of Guangdong, China, between autumn and winter of 2002. In February of 2003, it spread to Southeast Asia areas such as Taiwan, and at the end of March, the World Health Organization issued a warning to the world and officially named the disease SARS.

當年，隨著 SARS 在東南亞地區的爆發，臺灣成為了疫情災區，可由於臺灣與中國之間有著較為複雜的政治關係，早在 1971 年，因為中華人民共和國取得在聯合國中國代表權，臺灣作為中華民國政府被迫退出了聯合國及包括世界衛生組織在內的下屬機構，正式失去與世界衛生組織相互間的官方聯繫。

That year, following the outbreak of SARS in Southeast Asia, Taiwan was hit hard by the disease. Still, due to the complicated political relationship between Taiwan and China, as early as 1971, Taiwan, as the government of the Republic of China, was forced to withdraw from the United Nations and its subordinate agencies, including the World Health Organization, because the UN recognized the People's Republic of China as the government representing China. As a result, Taiwan lost the official link with the WHO.

也因此，臺灣沒有收到任何 SARS 爆發的疫情消息。

Consequently, Taiwan did not receive any information about the outbreak of SARS.

儘管在 1997 年開始，臺灣每年都會嘗試以不同名義重新參與世界衛生組織以及世界衛生大會，但均遭到 WHO 秘書處的拒絕。於是在 2003 年爆發的 SARS 疫情中，臺灣因為無法參與世界衛生組織，無法接收到最新防疫報告與防疫政策建議，同時又因中國以「於法不符，於理不容，於情不合」的理由進行打壓，因此臺灣便被國際視為「中國的一個省」，正式的失去了加入世界衛生組織的可能，並且無法獲得任何來自於世界衛生組織的醫療援助。

Taiwan has tried to rejoin the World Health Organization and the World Health Assembly in different names every year since 1997 but has always been rejected by the WHO Secretariat. In the outbreak of SARS in 2003, because Taiwan could not participate in the World Health Organization, it did not receive the latest epidemic prevention report and epidemic prevention policy recommendations. At the same time due to China's suppression on the grounds of "inconsistent with the law, unreasonable, inconsistent with the situation," Taiwan was regarded as "a province of China" by the international community, and formally lost the possibility of joining the World Health Organization, thus had no access to any medical assistance from the World Health Organization.

當時對抗 SARS 的戰爭，臺灣孤立無援。

In the combat with SARS, Taiwan was alone with no aid.

2003 年 4 月 24 日，臺灣台北和平醫院因 SARS 疫情突然爆發封院事件，是臺灣第一件因 SARS 感染而封院的事件。

April 24, 2003, the major outbreak of SARS in Taipei Municipal Hoping Hospital was the first hospital shutdown due to SARS infection In Taiwan.

2003 年 5 月 4 日，臺灣 SARS 疑似病例暴增，累計病例為 116 例、新增 14 例、疑似病例增加 82 例，為過去統計數的一倍。另外，臺灣整體通報人數已經達到 732 例，截至於當時國際標準時間 5 月 5 日 18 時，全球 SARS 確診與疑似病例共達 6,583 例，當時臺灣的確認與疑似確認病例人數，達到了全球的十分之一。

On May 4, 2003, cases of SARS seemed to have sharply increased in Taiwan, with 116 accumulated cases, and 14 new cases, 82 suspected cases, doubling the record before. Moreover, the total number of reported cases in Taiwan has reached 732. As of 18:00 on May 5, the international standard time, there were 6583 confirmed and suspected SARS cases in the world. At that time, the number of confirmed and suspected SARS cases in Taiwan reached one-tenth of that globally.

2003 年 7 月 5 日，世衛組織將臺灣從疫區中除名，至 7 月 30 日為止，臺灣隔離了共約 15 萬人。

On July 5, 2003, WHO removed Taiwan from the list of areas with recent local transmission of SARS, Taiwan has quarantined about 150000 people up to that time.

在這個孤立無援的情況下，由於臺灣無法在第一時間內獲得世界衛生組織的警告與相關的防疫醫療資源，為了生存，臺灣只好自行發展醫療技術，自行抗疫。

Being isolated with no aid, because Taiwan could not obtain the warning and relevant epidemic prevention medical resources from the World Health Organization in the first instance, to survive, Taiwan had to develop its medical technology and fight the epidemic independently.

至於這跟我們能在這次新冠肺炎有效抗疫有什麼關係？因為我可以很自豪的說：

As for how is this related to our effective combat against the coronavirus? It's because I can proudly say:

「為了這一天，我們的人民與政府已經準備了足足 17 年！」

"For this day, our people and government have been ready for 17 years!"

17 年前因為政治因素，臺灣成為了瘟疫孤島，從那個時候開始，存活便成為了臺灣人當時唯一的目標，為了活下來，人民與政府只好一同在孤立無援的世界瘟疫中找到生存的辦法。

Due to political issues, 17 years ago, Taiwan became an isolated island of the epidemic. Since that time, survival became the sole objective of Taiwanese people. In order to live, the people and the government had to work together to find a way to survive in a situation where there is no outside help, and they have to count on themselves.

套用 1993 年史蒂芬·史匹柏所導的〔侏儸紀公園〕中所說的一句話:「生命會找到自己的出路(Life will find its way out)。」

Quoting from the film Jurassic Park directed by Steven Spielberg, "Life will find its way out."

是的！我們存活下來了。

Yes! We lived.

臺灣身為一名在充滿血腥政治鬥爭下的犧牲者與求生者，我們不斷地尋找克服瘟疫的辦法，SARS 這個血淋淋的歷史教訓讓我們不忘防疫的精神，我們不斷地演練、不斷地求生，無論是否會造成瘟疫，我們都戰戰兢兢地看待每一個有可能會變成瘟疫的疾病。

As a victim and survivor in the bloody political struggle, Taiwan is continuously looking for ways to overcome the plague. The bloody historical lesson of SARS makes us not forget the spirit of epidemic prevention. We are constantly practicing and surviving, regardless of whether an epidemic will breakout, we are all wary of every disease that may turn into an epidemic.

被國際拋棄的這些年，我們預防、我們治療，我們之所以能在這次新冠肺炎的疫情中抗疫成功，只因為我們想生存，只因為我們不想再次因為一場瘟疫失去身邊的親友愛人，只因為我們不想再因為被世界拋棄而被迫孤軍奮戰。

In the years of being abandoned by the international community, we kept practicing prevention measures and treatments. The reason we can successfully combat the pandemic of COVID 19 is that we want to survive. After all, we don’t want to lose our family and friends once again due to a disease. We don’t want to be forced to fight alone, being abandoned by the world.

於是在這次的新冠肺炎疫情中，我們將能持續存活。

So in the outbreak of COVID 19, we will continue to survive.

在我寫這段文字的期間，我相信還有許多的人們正在為防疫而努力奮鬥，臺灣保持零確診優良紀錄的背後，是血淋淋的犧牲、是夾縫求生、是所有人的共同努力、是所有人互相支持的信念，在這個瘟疫肆虐的 2020 年，要存活的辦法就是要保持信念與持續警惕，別放棄繼續生存的想法，養精蓄銳，保持體力才有能力與新冠肺炎疫情持續對抗。

While I'm writing these words, I believe that many people are still struggling for pandemic prevention. Behind Taiwan's excellent record of zero confirmed cases lies the bloody sacrifice, the spirits to survive in a time of adversity, the joint efforts of all people and the belief that everyone would support each other. In 2020, the year rampaged by the pandemic, the way to survive is to keep faith and vigilance. Don't give up on the hope of surviving, only by keeping your strength can you continue with the combat with the coronavirus.

孤島求生

Survival on the Island of Isolation

在四處環海的孤島上我們只能生存

On an Island surrounded by sea, we could only survive on our own

臺灣於 2020 年 1 月 21 日確認出現首位新型冠狀病毒患者。

On January 21, 2020, Taiwan confirmed the first patient of coronavirus.

2020 年 1 月 23 日，世界衛生組織召開緊急會議，並在新冠肺炎疫情的報告確認臺灣通報的一個確診個案，然而在這次緊急會議中，臺灣並未在會議的邀請名單之中。

On January 23rd, 2020, the WHO called for an emergency meeting and confirmed a COVID-19 case reported by Taiwan in the report; however, in this emergency meeting, Taiwan was not included in the invitations list.

臺灣成為了唯一一個有移入個案而未獲世界衛生組織邀請的國家。

Taiwan became the only country with an imported case that has not been invited by the WHO.

世界衛生組織在新冠肺炎疫情的報告中，配合中華人民共和國蠻橫無理要求，不僅將臺灣列入中國之中，將臺灣及中華人民共和國在疫情地圖上標示為同一顏色，更在數日內多次更改臺灣的稱呼，先由「中國臺灣」改為「台北直轄市」，再改為「台北」，最後改為「台北及周圍地區」，有嚴重貶損臺灣的國家主權、地位及國格，有協助中國政府對臺灣繼續進行政治打壓之嫌疑。

In the WHO coronavirus report, to comply with China's unreasonable demands, it not only incorporated Taiwan in China but also marked Taiwan and People's Republic of China in the same colour on the epidemic map and changed the name of Taiwan several times within a few days. First, it was "Chinese Taiwan," then "Taipei Municipality," then back to "Taipei," and finally, "Taipei and its surrounding areas" seriously undermining Taiwan's sovereignty, status and national status. The WHO is suspected of assisting the Chinese government in its political suppression on Taiwan.

歷史的苦痛再度輪迴，臺灣又得像在 2003 年獨自面對 SARS 的瘟疫風暴一樣，再度被世界拋棄。

The pain of history repeats, Taiwan is abandoned by the world yet again, like how it faced the storm of the SARS epidemic alone in 2003.

幸好，面對這個嚴峻的狀況對我們來說已經不是第一次，由於我們過去有面對 SARS 的抗疫經驗，這次臺灣的疫情處理程序比過去更加提前且迅速，更有熱心的民眾於 2019 年 12 月 31 日，中國大陸湖北省武漢市的疫情爆發期間及時整理資訊並在臺灣的網路 PTT 論壇上發布，讓政府能更快速地看見這波疫情的發生，並提前做好防疫準備。

Fortunately, it's not the first time for us to face this grim situation. Because of our experience in fighting SARS in the past, Taiwan's pandemic handling procedures are more advanced and timelier than in the past. On December 31, 2019, an enthusiastic civilian even organized the information of the pandemic outbreak in Wuhan City, Hubei Province, China in time and released it on the Internet forum PTT in Taiwan, so that the government could see the happenings of the outbreak more quickly and prepare for it in advance.

同時，在臺灣發現瘟疫跡象的當天，臺灣的衛生福利部疾病管制署副署長於當天上午寄送電子郵件向中國疾控中心查證，並同時發放電子郵件至世界衛生組織的聯繫窗口。

At the same time, when signs of the disease were found in Taiwan, the deputy director of Center for Disease Control in Taiwan sent an email to Chinese Center for Disease Control and Prevention in China the contact window of the World Health

Organization for verification in the morning of the same day.

在臺灣寄送給世界衛生組織的郵件中，除了請教世界衛生組織相關的疫情資訊外，也特別提及到「非典型肺炎」、「病患已進行隔離治療」等瘟疫相關字眼，並強烈暗示此次瘟疫極有可能有人傳人的狀況發生。

In the email Taiwan sent to the WHO, other than inquiring the WHO about virus-related information, the email especially mentioned "atypical pneumonia," "patients have been isolated for treatment," and other virus-related words and strongly suggesting human-to-human transmission may be possible.

我們得到的回覆僅只表示「收到了」，便沒有後續的消息。

The only response we received was "received," with no subsequent response.

同時，為了有效傳達瘟疫發生的可能，臺灣中華民國外交部也請駐日內瓦辦事處與世界衛生組織秘書處聯繫，而我方仍只收到了「知道了！會轉給專家處理」的搪塞訊息，後續對瘟疫調查處理的結果及瘟疫造成的可能性傳播並未向世界公布。

At the same time, in order to adequately alert the possibility of the disease, the Ministry of Foreign Affairs of the Republic of China of Taiwan also requested the Geneva office to contact the Secretariat of the World Health Organization, but the message received was nothing but prevarication, "

"Oh, we will pass it to the related experts." The follow-up investigation results and the possible spread of the disease have not been disclosed to the world.

儘管臺灣面對國際的態勢如此嚴峻，但就像 1997 年一樣，我們並未放棄爭取加入國際並為國際貢獻的權力，雖說在 2017 年中國透過政治打壓致使臺灣再次未能獲得世界衛生大會的邀請函，但我們仍把握與世界交流的機會，並將臺灣擁有的技術、知識與資源持續地奉獻給各個國家，只因為我們秉持著一個信念：

Although Taiwan is facing such a difficult situation globally, just like in 1997, we have not given up our right to join the international community and contribute to the international community. Although China's political repression in 2017 prevented Taiwan from receiving the World Health Assembly's invitation again, we still seize the opportunity to communicate with the world and continue to dedicate the technology, knowledge, and resources possessed by Taiwan with various countries, only because we uphold the belief that:

「病毒不分國界，我們是世界的一員，全球防疫不應有缺口，全世界需要攜手合作，儘管我們被排除在世界衛生組織和聯合國之外，但我們仍願意分享專業、技術、資源及有關的防疫資訊與世界合作，共同度過這個難關。」

"Disease knows no borders, we are a part of the world, and there shouldn't be any gap in global disease prevention, the whole world needs to work together. Even though we have been excluded from the WHO and the UN, we are still willing

to share our expertise, technology, resources and relevant disease prevention information with the world to cooperate and overcome this difficulty."

而中國外交部在新冠肺炎疫情急劇升高期間，不僅沒有向臺灣分享疫情的資訊，還以中央政府自居進行政治操作與持續進行政治打壓，儘管臺灣對國際保持著共同合作抗疫的態度，但在 5 月 18 日第 73 屆 WHA 世界衛生大會線上會議召開時，臺灣仍未獲邀出席，不過我們並未放棄希望，儘管臺灣到目前為止仍未能參與國際性組織的抗疫活動，但我們仍獲得不少國家支持與效仿，達成更有效率的防疫措施。

During the rapid rise of COVID-19, the Chinese Ministry of Foreign Affairs not only did not share information on the pandemic with Taiwan, but also carried out political operations and continued political suppression in the name of the central government of China, and despite Taiwan maintains the attitude of cooperating with the international community against the pandemic. Taiwan was still not invited to the 73rd WHA World Health Assembly online meeting on May 18. Yet we did not give up hope. Although Taiwan has so far failed to participate in international organizations' anti-pandemic activities, we still received support and are followed by many countries in effective anti-pandemic measures.

如韓國也參考了我國對口罩發放的政策，宣布將提高徵收口罩的比例，推行「口罩實名制」，並實施與臺灣類似的 7 天買 2 片，依尾數分流購買等。
For example, South Korea took reference of our mask distribution policy, and announced that it would increase the proportion of masks to be collected, and implement mask-rationing plan, similar to that of Taiwan, where people can buy 2 masks in seven days, according to the end number of their ID.

由於臺灣在防疫初期執行了多項超前部署措施及後續應對

方案，在對抗疫情的期間臺灣開始在國際上獲得讚賞，我國並於 4 月 1 日給予世界各國醫療援助，如捐贈美國 200 萬片、歐洲國家 700 萬片口罩及邦交國 100 萬片口罩。

Since Taiwan implemented several advanced prevention measures and follow-up response plans in the early stage of pandemic prevention, Taiwan began to gain international appreciation while fighting the disease. On April 1, we also provided medical assistance to countries worldwide, such as donating 2 million masks to the United States, 7 million masks to European countries and 1 million masks to countries of diplomatic relations with Taiwan.

除此之外，臺灣也捐贈國產熱像體溫顯示儀 84 台與額溫槍等防疫物資，且在疫情期間，臺灣宜蘭當地民眾發起慈善募捐為疫情重災區的義大利捐贈將進 500 萬美元的醫療善款，並分享臺灣的電子檢疫系統與公開醫療設備「插管箱」的設計圖，讓有需要的國家可以更準確地追蹤確的診民眾接觸史，更持續讓我國的公私立醫院透過視訊方式提供各國相關的防疫經驗與技術。

Moreover, Taiwan also donated 84 domestic-made thermal image thermometers and forehead thermometers and other pandemic prevention supplies. During the outbreak, local people in Ilan, Taiwan, launched a fundraiser and donated US $5 million to Italy, the pandemic's hardest-hit area. The designs of Taiwan's digital fence technologies and medical equipment "Aerosol box" are also shared so that countries in need can more accurately track the patients' contact history. In Taiwan, public and private hospitals continue to provide relevant experience and technology of pandemic prevention in various countries through video exchanges.

儘管臺灣被排除於世界衛生組織和聯合國之外，但我們仍願意分享臺灣的防疫資源及過去對抗 SARS 的經驗，與世界各國合作，共同度過這道難關。

Although Taiwan is excluded from the World Health Organization and the United Nations, we are still willing to share Taiwan's pandemic prevention resources and experience in combating SARS, to cooperate with the countries worldwide to overcome this difficulty.

而我們之所以會為國際做這些事，是因為我們不希望自己曾經體會過的痛苦轉嫁到其他無辜的人身上，願意參與國際外交，是為了是能捍衛自己深愛的國家與促進國際間的交流，與世界一同走向自由與和平。

We are willing to do this for the world is we don't want the pain we have experienced to pass on to other innocent people. We are eager to participate in international diplomacy to defend our beloved country and promote international communication with the world towards freedom and peace.

反射神經 Reflective Nerves

過去的慘烈戰疫烙印在人們的心中

The bitter memories of past combat against the disease are branded in people's heart

2003 年臺灣因 SARS 隔離 15 萬人，2020 年臺灣持續零確診。

In 2003, Taiwan quarantined 150,000 people due to SARS. In 2020, Taiwan continues to have zero confirmed cases.

歷史的教訓造就了人民防疫的本能，除了 2003 年的 SARS 風波之外，臺灣在 1998 年也曾興起過一波腸病毒大流行，當時造成數十萬人感染，重症病例 405 人，更有 78 位以上病童因而致死。

The lessons of history have cultivated people's instincts for epidemic prevention. In addition to the SARS storm in 2003,

Taiwan also had a wave of enterovirus pandemics in 1998, which caused hundreds of thousands of infections at that time, 405 severe cases, and more than 78 children killed.

由於腸病毒的傳染多因成人自外面帶回，經由接觸或飛沫傳染的方式感染家中幼童造成，因此臺灣當時為確實落實防疫，故在電視、報章雜誌等大眾傳播媒體宣傳勤洗手的習慣，甚至現在臺灣大多數公民現在都還記得當時政府宣傳「**濕、搓、沖、捧、擦**」這五大洗手口訣。

Enterovirus infections are mostly caused by adults who brought the virus back from outside and transmitted them to young children at home by contact or droplet infection. Therefore, to effectively implement epidemic prevention in Taiwan, the habit of washing hands frequently was promoted in the mass media such as the TV, newspapers and magazines. Even now, most Taiwan citizens still remember the five major hand-washing steps the government promoted **"wet, rub, flush, hold, and rub."**

先不說臺灣時不時就會爆發的一些季節性傳染病，光是腸病毒與 SARS 這兩項曾經特別嚴重的傳染病經驗便使得臺灣人特別注重衛生保健習慣，甚至大多臺灣人在生病時會常態性的戴口罩以阻絕病毒的傳播，這也是我們臺灣人能在新冠肺炎疫情爆發初期，人民能快速配合政府部署防疫的關鍵原因。

Not mentioning the seasonal infectious diseases that break out in Taiwan from time to time, the experience of the two particularly infectious diseases, enterovirus and SARS, has made Taiwanese pay special attention to hygiene habits. Many people in Taiwan are in the habit of wearing a mask when they are sick to avoid transmission. Wearing masks to prevent the spread of the virus is a crucial reason we Taiwanese can quickly cooperate with the government to enforce epidemic prevention in the early stage of the outbreak of the COVID-19.

當然，除了過往的防疫經驗之外，也不得不歸功於臺灣有一項優良的醫療政策，這個政策不僅讓我們臺灣公民在看醫生的時候都不用花到什麼錢，甚至連因為緊急情況況不得不在國外就醫時，我們還有「海外就醫」的補助來補貼國外就診的高額費用。

Of course, in addition to the experience of past epidemic prevention, the sound medical policy in Taiwan which not only saves us Taiwanese citizens from spending almost any money when seeing doctors but also subsidize us for “overseas medical treatment” in emergencies where we have no choice but to seek medical aid abroad, is another key factor.

回來在臺灣看醫生這件事，在臺灣看醫生究竟有多便宜呢？只要你是台灣公民，大多數有在臺灣健保補貼範圍中的疾病只需要 5-15 美金之間就能被解決，之所以能靠這匪夷所思的價格完成治療，一方面是因為過去瘟疫所留下的慘痛經驗導致，另一部分則是歸功於臺灣健全的健保制度。

When it comes to seeing a doctor in Taiwan, how affordable is it to see a doctor in Taiwan? As long as you are a Taiwanese citizen, most of the Taiwan health insurance subsidy conditions can be covered, and the citizen only has to pay between 5-15 US dollars. The treatment can be completed at this incredible price partly because of the painful experience brought by past plague, partly due to Taiwan's sound health insurance system.

臺灣的健保制度全稱為全民健康保險，概念起源於 1986 年 5 月臺灣行政院核定的**中華民國臺灣經濟長期展望**。其中它提到 2000 年將計畫為全民健保的開辦目標年，這也是我國官方首次明確指出健保的實施概念。

Taiwan's health insurance system is called the National Health Insurance. The concept originated from the **long-term outlook of the Republic of China's Taiwanese economy** approved by the Taiwan Executive Yuan in May 1986. It mentions that the plan will be set as the target year for health insurance for all in 2000, which is also the first time that my country's officials have pointed out the concept of health insurance implementation.

而後，在 1988 年，行政院經建會專責規畫小組著手於全民健康保險的執行規劃，並完成全民健康保險規劃報告。1990 年 7 月，行政院衛生署接手規劃全民健康保險。1991 年 2 月衛生署成立全民健康保險規劃小組，進行細節討論作業。
Then, in 1988, the Special Planning Group of the Economic Construction Committee of the Executive Yuan set out to implement the plan for implementing the National Health Insurance and completed the National Health Insurance Planning Report. In July 1990, the Health Department of the Executive Yuan took over universal health insurance planning. In February 1991, the Department of Health established the National Health Insurance Planning Group to conduct detailed discussion operations.

我國全民健保原定於 2000 年實施，後再經官方多次決議後提前至 1995 年實施。同時，在 2003 年 SARS 疫情爆發的期間臺灣健保局推行了全民健保卡全面 IC 卡化的政策，讓所有有就醫紀錄的臺灣人能將過往就醫狀況整合在一張卡片的晶片裡，並在每次看診時上傳雲端伺服器，這不僅能提升醫生的診療正確率，還更方便臺灣人看醫生的流程。

After many official discussions, the country's National Health Insurance, initially scheduled to be implemented in 2000, moved to 1995. During the SARS outbreak in 2003, the Taiwan Health Insurance Bureau implemented a comprehensive IC card policy for all health insurance cards. All Taiwanese with medical records can integrate past medical conditions into the card's chip, which uploads to the cloud server in every hospital visit. It significantly improves the accuracy of doctors' diagnosis and treatment, making seeing a doctor easier for Taiwanese citizens.

另外，臺灣在 2013 年 7 月的時候也建立了以病人為中心的健保雲端藥歷系統，提供特約醫事服務機構的醫師在臨床處置、開立處方時及藥師用藥諮詢時，可以即時查詢病人過去 3 個月的用藥紀錄，避免重複用藥的情形發生，提升用藥安全及品質，讓病人只需攜帶健保卡，支付 5-15 美金，並向醫生說明清楚疾病狀況後就能享受到精確有效的醫療服務。

Moreover, in July 2013, Taiwan also established a patient-centric health care cloud medical prescription system, which enables physicians of medical service institutions to check patients' medical records in the past three months during clinical treatment to avoid repeated medication, improve safety and quality. Patients simply have to carry a health insurance card, pay 5-15 US dollars, and explain to the doctor their symptoms clearly, and they can enjoy accurate and effective medical treatment services.

就是因為有這些明確的醫療政策與完善的健保相關措施，也使得臺灣人在每當身邊的親朋好友生病時總會這樣問：

Because of these clear medical policies and comprehensive healthcare-related measures, Taiwanese people will always ask the following questions whenever their relatives and friends get sick:

「你去看醫生了沒？多喝點水。」

“Have you seen a doctor? Drink more water.”

更直接的人則會這樣說：

「感冒要戴口罩啊！我可不想被你傳染啊！」

Some people will even say bluntly:

“Wear a mask when you get a cold! I don’t want to catch it from you!”

從上述兩句話來針對臺灣人應對疾病的行為邏輯判斷，或許是因為過去 SARS 的影響，導致臺灣人民非常害怕生病或被身邊的人傳染，另一方面也可以體現出臺灣人對疾病的應對處理方式抱持著謹慎且採較有效率的方式態度（當然！這也跟在臺灣看醫生很便宜有很大的關係）。

From the above two sentences, we could tell that the logic of Taiwanese people’s behavioural response to disease may be due to the impact of SARS in the past, which caused the Taiwanese people to be terrified of getting sick or being infected by people around them. On the other hand, it also shows Taiwanese people's response to disease is cautious and more efficient (of course! This is also related to the fact that it is very affordable to see a doctor in Taiwan).

當然！這種行為模式是建立在從小到大的健康教育環境與優秀的健保制度下才能被塑造的，若是缺少了其中一項，估計臺灣現在也不見得能在防疫的基礎下做出零確診的成蹟。

Of course! Two factors lead to such a behavioural model, the health education environment, and the excellent health insurance system in which Taiwanese people have experienced since they were little. If either factor is missing, it is possible Taiwan would not have reached zero diagnosis record.

防毒面具 Gas Mask

想要隔絕毒氣你需要一張防毒面具

To block out poisonous gas, you need a gas mask

疫情期間，為了減少被外界病毒感染的可能，世界各地的民眾在外出期間開始陸續戴上口罩。也因如此，大多數國家的民眾也已經開始逐漸適應並認同戴口罩能有效防疫這個事實。

During the pandemic, to reduce the possibility of being infected by outside viruses, people worldwide began wearing medical masks one after another during outings. Thus, people in most countries have gradually adapted to and agree that wearing masks can effectively prevent the epidemic.

但在疫情嚴重爆發之前，多數國家的民眾並未有攜帶口罩的習慣，這也導致多數歐美國家無法理解像臺灣這種一有傳染病跡象，甚至只要空氣品質下降便會集體帶上口罩的國家，這種輕易就戴上口罩的行為對多數將戴口罩認定為「**生重病**」或「**前往醫院**」的人來說無疑是非常「**過激**」的。

Before the pandemic outbreak, people in most countries did not have the habit of wearing masks. Thus, most European and American countries fail to understand a country like Taiwan, where people start wearing masks when there are signs of infectious diseases, or even when the air quality declines. Such a natural tendency of putting on a mask is undoubtedly seen as **"excessive"** for most people who think only people who are **"seriously ill"** or **"going to the hospital"** should wear a mask.

除了前幾個小節提到臺灣因為過去曾面臨過多次較嚴重的傳染病事件導致臺灣人普遍能接受日常戴口罩的原因之外，或許就該提到臺灣過去興起的哈日文化了。

In addition to the reasons mentioned in the previous subsections that Taiwan has faced many serious infectious diseases in the past, which made it generally acceptable for

Taiwanese to wear masks daily, perhaps it is time to mention the Japanophile culture that Taiwan has developed in the past.

所謂臺灣的哈日文化是指崇拜、複製日本流行文化的文化行為，在具體解釋臺灣哈日文化的興起原因之前，我們先來解釋為什麼這個文化能讓臺灣人使用口罩普及的原因。
The so-called Japanophile culture in Taiwan refers to the cultural behaviour of worshiping and copying Japanese popular culture. Before specifically explaining the rise of Japanophile culture in Taiwan, let's first explain why this culture can make wearing masks popular in Taiwan.

早在新冠肺炎興起之前，日本就有不少人有外出戴口罩的習慣，**對大多數的日本人來說戴口罩就像是夏天戴墨鏡、冬天圍圍巾一樣的稀鬆平常**，那為什麼戴口罩對日本人來說是如此的「常態」呢？
Before the outbreak of the COVID-19, many people in Japan had the habit of wearing masks when going out. For most

Japanese people, wearing masks is like wearing sunglasses in summer and scarves in winter, so why wear masks? Why is it the "norm" for the Japanese?

第一點源自於日本的職場文化，在大多數國家的職場文化中，生病請病假、不想工作請特休是再正常不過的一件事情，但對日本人來說上述這個職場文化是不存在的。

The first reason stems from the Japanese workplace culture. In most countries' workplace culture, it is reasonable to ask for leave when one is sick or does not want to work or want to take special breaks, but for Japanese people, the above workplace culture is non-existing.

在日本，病假與特休是合併再一起計算的，也就是說，日本人的職場文化中根本就沒有所謂的病假，畢竟誰會將寶貴的假期浪費在生病這件事情上面呢？

In Japan, sick leave and special holidays are combined and calculated together; that is to say, there is no such thing as sick leave in Japanese workplace culture. After all, who will waste precious vacations on sickness?

正因如此，多數日本人在工作日期間生病時也會前往工作地點工作，但由於日本的禮節文化使得該國國民非常顧慮周遭的想法，所以為了預防自己將傳染病傳染給別人，他們便會戴上口罩以隔絕病毒。

For this reason, most Japanese people still go to work when they are sick during workdays. However, due to Japan's courtesy culture, its citizens are very concerned about the opinions of those around them, so to prevent themselves from transmitting infectious diseases to others, they wear a mask to isolate the virus.

第二點則是源自於日本當地的氣候了，日本在冬季時氣候非常乾燥，容易引起流鼻血及嘴唇乾裂的現象，既不雅觀又不舒適，且在初春時節許多患有花粉症的人們容易吸入飄散在空氣中的花粉，也因此只好養成戴口罩的習慣。

The second reason stems from the local climate of Japan. In winter, Japan has an arid environment, which is prone to cause nosebleeds and dry lips. It is unsightly and uncomfortable. In the early spring, many people with hay fever. It is easy to inhale the pollen floating in the air, so people developed the habit of wearing a mask.

這時對臺灣有點理解的人可能會覺得有些奇怪，臺灣既沒有日本的職場文化，也沒有氣候乾澀的問題（**臺灣為介於熱帶及亞熱帶氣候的國家**），那為什麼一模仿起日本文化後便開始引發了全民戴口罩的風潮呢？
At this point, people with a little understanding of Taiwan may find it strange. Taiwan has neither a Japanese workplace culture nor the problem of dry climate **(Taiwan is a country between tropical and subtropical climates).** Why did it start imitating Japanese culture and triggered the wave of people wearing masks?

那就是上述這些原因並非完全是日本人會這麼常態性會戴口罩的真正原因，主要他們會這麼常態性戴口罩是因文化形態的「**禮節包袱**」導致，以下我便具體解釋兩個關鍵的原因。

That is because the above reasons are not exactly why it's a norm for Japanese people to wear masks. The main reason why they wear masks is the "burden of etiquette" in cultural forms. I will explain two key reasons specifically.

第一點是由禮節文化導致的社交障礙問題，日本禮節文化最早的起源可以追朔自古代中國，過去古代中國的聖賢曾說：「君子之交淡若水」，這句話用比較容易理解的方式來說就是，身為一個有禮貌的人，就算是面對好朋友，也要點到為止。

The first point is the problem of social barriers caused by etiquette culture. The earliest origin of Japanese etiquette culture can trace back to ancient China. In the past, ancient China's sages once said: "The friendship between gentlemen is light." A simple way to understand it is, as a polite person, even when facing a good friend, you have to behave appropriately.

相比於西方國家較親暱的肢體接觸與較充滿溫度的禮節，多數受到古代中國影響的東方國家多保留著保持社交距離及冷靜、沉著，對事情表現淡然的禮節文化。
Compared with the more intimate physical contact and warmer etiquette in Western countries, most Eastern countries were influenced by ancient China and retain a culture of etiquette where people maintain social distance with a calm, rational, and composed attitude.

這也讓日本人會將口罩當作是圍巾戴關鍵原因，因為戴上口罩之後周遭的其他人就會自動與自己保持距離（儘管是東方國家，多數人仍會將戴口罩聯想成「患上感冒」的聯想)，於是透過這個行為就可以減少過多的社交，且口罩能遮住部分表情，這讓日本人能更輕鬆地保持冷靜沉著的態度與人相處。

This also makes the Japanese see wearing masks as wearing scarves (even though in eastern countries, most people still associate wearing masks as "catching a cold"). When wearing a mask, other people around will automatically keep a distance so that this behaviour can reduce excessive social interaction. Masks can cover part of the expression, making it easier for the Japanese to maintain a calm and composed attitude toward people.

另外一個原因則是因為美觀了，很多時候日本人會因為下半後去居酒屋報到的職場文化而熬夜在居酒屋喝酒，這也導致隔日上班宿醉的狀態變成了常態，而多數有宿醉經驗的人肯定知道，宿醉時不光是頭欲炸裂，更會面容憔悴（因為起床之後就趕著上班沒時間化妝或刮鬍子，再加上熬夜導致內分泌失調而臉上冒痘），這時口罩便成為了「遮羞布」，除了能遮擋面容憔悴的自己，更能讓其他人有意無意地產生社交距離，遮掩自己宿醉的事實。

Another reason is aesthetic. In many cases, the Japanese will stay up and drink in the izakaya due to the workplace culture of going to an izakaya in the second half of the evening, which causes hangover at work the next day to become the norm. Most people who had hangovers before must know that it is not only about having terrible migraines but also haggard-looking faces (having no time to put on makeup or shave after getting up and rushing to work. Moreover, staying up late may have caused endocrine disorders and acne on their faces). Then the mask becomes the "shame cloth," which could cover their haggard face and allow others to intentionally or unintentionally create a social distance and cover up the fact of their hangover.

當然！除了職場文化之外，日本多數年輕女性都會有化妝的習慣，但因為很多時候需要早起上學上班，因此便會很常出現因為要趕著出門而無暇打扮的狀況，這時口罩這個「遮羞布」便變成了美顏神器，因此這也讓戴口罩這個行為在日本變得相當普遍。

Of course! In addition to workplace culture, most young women in Japan have the habit of wearing makeup. However, because they often need to get up early for school or work, they often encounter situations where they have no time to dress up because they have to rush out. At this time, the mask becomes the "shame cloth". It's a beauty enhancement tool, so the behaviour of wearing a mask has become quite common in Japan.

上述的兩點同時也是我認為口罩在臺灣哈日文化盛行的期間能真正風靡全台的關鍵原因，而之所以臺灣會有哈日文化盛行的原因則是，一方面臺灣在 1895 年至 1945 年間受到日本的殖民統治時吸收了一定量的日本禮節文化，這使得部分人對模仿日本文化的流行產生了認同感，一方面則是因為早期臺灣大量播放充斥著日本文化的電視節目、動漫、電玩導致。

The above two points are also the key reason why masks

became popular during the prevalence of Japanophile culture in Taiwan. Japanophile culture is prevalent in Taiwan because, on the one hand, Taiwan was influenced by Japan during the colonial rule of Japan, a certain amount of Japanese etiquette culture was absorbed, which made some people identify with the trend of imitating Japanese culture. On the other hand, it was caused by a large number of TV programs, anime, and video games that were full of Japanese culture in early Taiwan.

同時，許多少女認為口罩擁有遮擋面容甚至是美化面容的效果，光是這點就讓非常多的少年少女競相推廣哈日文化，在當時臺灣哈日文化盛行的期間，戴口罩可是被不少少年少女認為是追隨流行時尚尖端的表現呢！
Simultaneously, many girls think that masks have the effect of covering faces or even beautifying faces. This alone has made many young girls compete in promoting the Japanophile culture. When the Japanophile culture was prevalent in Taiwan, wearing masks was considered by many young girls as a sign of

following cutting edge fashion!

現在在臺灣，口罩不僅成為了我國國民日常必備的戰疫物資，政府更砸下重本**委託臺灣在地各個口罩生產廠商加大產量**，讓口罩成為防疫關鍵資源，更推行**口罩實名制**，不讓民眾因為過度恐慌造成囤貨，導致未能及時購買的民眾喪失防疫的可能。

Now in Taiwan, masks have become a daily necessary epidemic material for citizens, but the government has also invested heavily in **entrusting various mask manufacturers in Taiwan to increase production.** Masks are a vital resource for epidemic prevention. It enforces a mask rationing system to prevent the public from falling into stockpiling panic leading to hoarding of goods, which may cause some people to be unable to purchase pandemic prevention materials in time.

同時這也使得我國從原先的口罩進口國，瞬間晉升為**全球第二大口罩生產國**，甚至還創立了**口罩預購 APP**，讓人們不用外出排隊搶口罩，輕鬆透過網路下單直接購買，讓人民不再因為口罩的匱乏而冒著群聚感染的風險到處搶口罩。

At the same time, it made Taiwan instantly become the **second-largest mask producer in the world**, and even created a **pre-order mask app**, so that people can easily place orders directly through the Internet without going out to queue for masks. Hence, citizens no longer need to fight for buying masks everywhere because of the scarcity of masks and risk cluster infection.

超前部署 Advanced Deployment
事前的規劃永遠都是最安全的選項
Early planning is always the safest choice

若是有人在疫情爆發前跟你說，有個國家在疫情爆發之前就開始組建疫情指揮中心，並陸續傳達多項防疫辦法與補助措施，且於每日 14:00 分時及時向全國民眾彙報即時的戰疫資訊，你或許會覺得這個國家肯定是瘋了，又或者是國家預算太多需要被消耗一下。

If someone tells you before the outbreak, a country started setting up an epidemic command center before the outbreak, followed by a series of epidemic prevention measures and subsidies, and promptly report to the citizen of the country at 14:00 every day the updates of epidemic information, you may think that this country must be crazy or it has too much budget that needs to be consumed.

但在疫情爆發的期間，若有人對你說上述的這些話，你肯定會想知道是哪個國家這麼前瞻，現在是不是還可以去那個國家避避風頭。

However, during the epidemic outbreak, if someone said these words to you, you would want to know which country has such foresight and whether it is still possible to go to that country to keep off the wind.

上述所說的國家就是臺灣。

The country mentioned above is Taiwan.

2020 年 1 月 20 日，因應國際已有多起嚴重特殊傳染性肺炎案例，國家衛生指揮中心針對新冠肺炎開設「嚴重特殊傳染性肺炎中央流行疫情指揮中心」。

On January 20, 2020, in response to many cases of severe special infectious pneumonia in the world, the National Health Command Center established the "Severe Special

Infectious Pneumonia Central Epidemic Command Center" for COVID-19.

臺灣在過去曾有多次傳染病的抗疫經驗，從過去曾經發生的腸病毒、SARS 等多項傳染病及各種季節性傳染病中，我們都很清楚臺灣成立中央流行疫情指揮中心的原因，但 2020 年 1 月 20 日這個時間點成立的「嚴重特殊傳染性肺炎中央流行疫情指揮中心」就令人匪夷所思了，如果你有仔細看前面幾個章節你就知道，臺灣第一起案例可是 1 月 21 日後才出現的啊！

In the past, Taiwan has had many experiences in fighting infectious diseases. From the enteric viruses, SARS and other infectious diseases and various seasonal infectious diseases that occurred in the past, we are well aware of the reasons for establishing the Central Epidemic Command Center. However, the "Severe Special Infectious Pneumonia Central Epidemic Command Center" was established on January 20, 2020. If you look carefully at the previous subsections, you will know that the first case of COVID-19 in Taiwan was January 21, after the Center was established!

看到這裡你或許會覺得，臺灣這個國家未免也太未卜先知了吧！連還沒發生的事情都可以提前預料到，並快速做出應對措施。

Seeing this, you might think that Taiwan is a prophet, foreseeing incidents that haven't happened yet in advance, and take quick response measures!

原來，之所以能未卜先知的原因還是源於臺灣過去 SARS 的防疫經驗，過去的防疫經驗不僅讓我們對可能發生的傳染病更加謹慎，也更知道遇到這種可能性會發生的瘟疫事件要怎麼妥善處理。

It turns out that the reason the disease could be predicted was due to Taiwan's past SARS epidemic prevention experience. Previous experience in epidemic prevention made us more cautious about possible infectious diseases and knew how to face the possibility of a virus outbreak and handle it properly.

再加上我國於 2019 年 12 月 31 日時就有網民提前爆料，中國大陸湖北省武漢市有疑似過去 SARS 傳染病爆發的消息，且我方政府為求慎重，不僅及時向世界衛生組織與中國中央確認消息，雖然對方似乎也沒有明確表達確實有此事發生，但我方仍不畏可能發生的政治打壓，提前針對武漢直航入境班機進行登機檢驗，並主動評估旅客健康情形與加強防疫宣導。

What's more, as early as December 31, 2019, a Taiwanese netizen broke the news of suspected news of a SARS-like infectious disease outbreak in Wuhan City, Hubei Province, China, and our government, to be cautious, contacted the WHO and China government for confirmation. Although neither party clearly expressed that this has happened, our government still enacted boarding inspection of direct flights from Wuhan, unafraid of possible political suppression, and took the initiative to assess passenger health and strengthen anti-epidemic declaration guides.

這也是為什麼臺灣在 1 月 21 日確認出現首位新型冠狀病毒患者後，病例增加的數成長比其他各國更為緩慢，且近乎未出現社區感染的關鍵原因。

This is also the key reason why the number of cases increased much slower than that of other countries after Taiwan confirmed the emergence of the first COVID-19 patient on January 21. There is almost no cluster infection.

後來，在三月多期間，新冠肺炎疫情的興起讓全世界引起了翻天覆地的變化，西方國家陸續「封國」、義大利死於新冠肺炎的人數超過中國大陸（雖然至今我們仍不是很清楚中國大陸的確切病例數）、西、德、美、法等國家的確診數則競相擠進了「萬人俱樂部」，甚至各國的股價也呈現溜滑梯向下的趨勢。

Later, during March, the COVID-19 pandemic rise has shaken the world, causing drastic changes. Western countries enforced "lockdown" one after another. Italy has more people who died of COVID-19 than mainland China (although we still do not know very well the exact number of confirmed COVID-19 cases in mainland China). Spain, Germany, America, France and other countries have entered the "10,000 Club", and even the stock prices of different countries have shown a downward trend on the slide.

而臺灣也不免俗的在這點與國際接軌。在當時，由於各國感染人數暴增，且臺灣尚未對其他國家採取班機停飛的政策，致使我國境外感染人數暴增，**從原先總感染數的五十二例增加到一三五例**，成長將近一倍，這也讓我國開始意識到，是時候該採取更「超前」的計畫了。

And Taiwan is inevitably in line with the international trend. At the time, the number of infections in various countries skyrocketed, and Taiwan had not adopted a policy of grounding flights from abroad, resulting in a surge in the number of infections from outside of Taiwan, **which increased from 53 cases to 135 cases**, which is almost double the amount of the initial number. This also made our country realize that it is time to adopt a more "advanced" plan.

當時，除了開始對各地航班進行**停飛政策**與推出**境外歸國隔離 14 天**等防疫政策外，為了因應未來新冠肺炎疫情擴散對全球造成的經濟衝擊，我國總統召集行政院正副院長及相關部會首長、國安會秘書長和諮詢委員緊急召開國安高層會議，雖說因我國防疫的超前部署國內疫情管控良好，但為因應疫情未來可能會造成的經濟衝擊，我國規劃了以下的計畫：

At that time, in addition to the **policy of grounding flights** and the launching of **14-day quarantine policy for people coming back from overseas,** to cope with the future economic impact on the world caused by the spread of the COVID-19, our President convened the deputy president of the Executive Yuan and the heads of relevant ministries. The Secretary-General of the National Security Council and the Advisory Committee urgently held a high-level meeting of the National Security

Council. Although the domestic epidemic situation was well controlled due to our nation's advanced deployment, in response to the economic impact that the epidemic may cause in the future, the government made the following plans:

一、針對因應受衝擊的產業提供 600 億的防疫紓困特別預算。

1. A special budget of NT $ 60 billion for epidemic prevention and relief will be provided for industries subject to the impact.

二、政府各部門既有預算及基金移緩濟急，除上述 600 億的紓困預算之外，緊急挪移政府預算及他項基金的支出，約有近 400 億經費可投入紓困與振興計畫。

2. All government departments move their original budgets and funds to the emergency relief budget. In addition to the aforementioned $0 billion relief budget and the spending of other government budgets and funding, there are almost

NT$40 billion of the budget put into relief and revitalization plan.

三、除持續前瞻基礎建設計畫進度外，就公共建設、政府採購、與包含長照幼托等公共服務的部分，以及國防產業及相關採購等，加大加速進行，以最高的效率、最短的時間落實各項擴大內需計畫。

3. In addition to continuing with the progress of advanced basic infrastructure, we will increase public work speed, government procurement, public services including long-term child care, and defence industry and related procurement, with the highest efficiency and the shortest time. Implement various plans to expand domestic demand.

四、除了公部門投資加速之外，全力協助民間加速投資，確實執行台商回流及投資臺灣方案，全力協助企業排除投資障礙，維繫民間投資動能及總體經濟活力。

4. In addition to accelerating investment in the public sector, we will fully assist the private sector in accelerating investment, ensuring implementation of the plan for Taiwanese businessmen to return and invest in Taiwan, and fully assist companies in removing investment barriers to maintain private investment momentum and overall economic vitality.

五、雖說臺灣經濟尚屬良好，但為避免疫情變化造成的心理層面影響，讓我國財政部、金管會、中央銀行等各部會密切觀察國際金融市場，全力維持匯市穩定與股市動能。

5. Although Taiwan's economy is relatively good, in order to avoid the psychological impact caused by changes caused by the pandemic, various ministries such as the Ministry of Finance, the Financial Management Commission, and the Central Bank of my country will carefully observe the international financial market and strive to maintain the stability of the foreign exchange market and the momentum of the stock market.

從上述在三月期間宣布的**「更超前部署」**計畫中我們可以看出來，臺灣在因多次抗疫下的經驗擁有了更前瞻的防疫視野，不僅可以提前看出疫情會爆發的徵兆，更提前預防之後可能會發生的金融危機，並透過完善的紓困補助制度來安定民心。

From the above-mentioned "**even more advanced deployment**" plan announced in March, we can see that Taiwan has a more forward-looking perspective on epidemic prevention because of its experience in fighting many epidemics. It can see the signs of an outbreak in advance and prevent the financial crises that may occur afterward and restore public confidence through a comprehensive relief system.

只能說，在這艱困的抗疫期間，身為一名臺灣人真的是一件非常幸福的事情，不僅國家有個能針對疫情影響提出全方位部署政策的戰疫指揮中心，更能公開地向民眾宣達正確的防疫資訊與防疫進度，並提供相對應的資源讓人民更有餘力與瘟疫進行對抗，讓人民不會因為疫情未知的恐懼而放棄希望。

I have to say that during this challenging pandemic combating period, being a Taiwanese is truly a blessing. The country has an epidemic command center that can propose a comprehensive prevention policy in response to the impact of the epidemic and openly publicize the correct epidemic prevention information and epidemic prevention progress to the people. Moreover, provide corresponding resources to make the people have more strength to fight against the virus so that they will not give up hope due to fear of uncertainty brought by the pandemic.

寫到這裡，我也希望能藉由自己的文字與臺灣大眾們的努力，一邊向世界各國推廣臺灣有效地防疫政策，一邊整理要如何根據自身的國情狀況訂定適合自己國民的防疫規則，並希望我們的宣傳能讓各國的人們看見且能影響周遭的人，讓他們知道目前的狀況雖然嚴峻，但仍不可以放棄抗疫希望，並期許各國政府能推出有效的防疫方案，讓人民脫離疫情的水深火熱之中。

When I write here, I hope that through my words and the Taiwanese people's efforts, I could let the people of all countries in the world know about Taiwan's effective epidemic prevention policies. And if applicable, they could adapt our strategies according to their nation's conditions to formulate their own pandemic prevention plans. We hope that this will allow people from all countries to see and affect those around them, letting them know that although the current situation is severe, they still have hope in defeating the pandemic. Furthermore, we hope the governments of various countries can launch effective anti-pandemic policies to save people from the sufferings of the epidemic.

護臺灣、助世界

臺灣能幫忙，而且臺灣正在幫忙

Taiwan can help
and Taiwan is helping

第二章
Chapter 2

臺灣是什麼

What is Taiwan

地球之島 An Island on earth
這個地方有著全世界的氣候與美景
This place has the best climate and views in the world

臺灣泛指為臺灣本島、澎湖列島、金門群島、馬祖列島、東沙群島、烏丘列嶼、南沙群島的太平島、中洲礁、釣魚臺列嶼及臺灣其離島等周圍海域的島群，是位於亞洲東部，居於東北亞和東南亞交會處的一個島嶼國家。

Taiwan generally refers to the island groups in the surrounding waters such as Taiwan's main island, Penghu Islands, Kinmen Islands, Matsu Islands, Dongsha Islands, Uchulieu Island, Nansha Islands, Taiping Island, Zhongzhou Reef, Diaoyutai Islands, and Taiwan's outlying islands, and more. It's an island country residing at the intersection of Northeast Asia and Southeast Asia.

臺灣地理環境四面環海，**位置約位於東經 120 度至 122 度，北緯 22 度至 25 度之間，總面積約為 36,188** 平方公里，東接菲律賓海、西與歐亞大陸相望、南濱巴士海峽，北接東海。

The sea surrounds the geographical environment of Taiwan, and the **location of Taiwan is about 120 degrees to 122 degrees east longitude, 22 degrees to 25 degrees north latitude, with a total area of about 36,188 square kilometers**, east to the Philippine Sea, west to Eurasia, south to the bus strait, north to the East China Sea

由於四面環海的特色，臺灣孕育了各色的海岸地形，其中可分為岬角與海灣相間的北部岩岸、海岸線平直單調的西部沙岸、珊瑚礁地形為主的南部珊瑚礁海岸、山地和海洋相鄰的東部斷層海岸，因此許多觀光客會前往臺灣各個海岸及離島，享受珊瑚礁的島嶼風情、垂釣及浮潛的樂趣。

Being surrounded by the sea, Taiwan features a wide range of coastal terrains, which can be divided into the rocky northern shore between the headland and the bay, the flat and monotonous coastline of the western sand shore, the southern coral reef coast dominated by coral reef terrain, mountain and ocean, and the eastern fault of the coast. Thus many tourists will go to various beaches and islands in Taiwan to enjoy the coral reefs, island style, fishing and snorkeling.

在地勢方面，臺灣的地勢東高西低，由地殼擠壓抬升而形成主要的地形有山地、丘陵、盆地、台地、平原，其中我國的山脈**以高山聳立聞名國際**。

In terms of topography, Taiwan is high in the east and low in the west. The primary terrain formed by the crustal extrusion is mountains, hills, basins, terraces, and plains. Among them, **the mountains in the country are famous for their height internationally.**

臺灣的山脈以中央山脈為主體，地勢高峻陡峭，且因島嶼面積小，使得地勢格外高聳陡峭。在短短數十公里內，從海平面拔高近 3,000～4,000 公尺，形成雄偉壯麗的高山深谷地景，是國際有名的「高山島嶼國家」。

The Central Mountain Range dominates the mountain range in Taiwan, and the terrain is high and steep. Due to the small area of the island, it makes the terrain extremely high and steep. Within a few tens of kilometers, it has risen nearly 3,000 to 4,000 meters from the sea level, forming a magnificent mountain scenery with high mountains and deep valleys. It is an internationally renowned "alpine island country."

在臺灣，三千公尺以上的高山比比皆是，其原因是臺灣的地塊較為活躍，地殼快速抬升，**3,000 公尺以上的高峰多達 200 多座**，其中以玉山最高，達 3,952 公尺，為東亞鄰近地區最高峰。另有中央山脈、玉山山脈、雪山山脈、阿里山山脈與海岸山脈，共同形成臺灣的五大山地，是臺灣大多數的登山客都會去朝聖的觀光景點，且因地理資源的豐沛，臺灣擁有許多特殊地形及奇特的地理景觀。

In Taiwan, it's common to see high mountains that are over 3,000 meters. The reason is that Taiwan's plots are more active, and the crust is rapidly rising. There are more than 200 peaks above 3,000 meters, of which Yushan is the highest, reaching 3,952 meters. It is the highest peak in East Asia. The Central Mountain Range, Yushan Mountain Range, Snow Mountain Range, Alishan Mountain Range, and Coastal Mountain Range form the five mountainous areas of Taiwan, where most mountaineers in Taiwan will go as scenic pilgrimage spots. Because of the abundant geographical resources, Taiwan has many unique terrains and peculiar geographical landscapes.

除了高山之外，臺灣還有非常多優美的海岸風光，從北算起擁有各類特殊海岸地形的東北角暨宜蘭海岸國家風景區、北海岸及觀音山國家風景區，山青水秀、大藍海深，廣闊藍天便是此地段的特色。

In addition to the high mountains, Taiwan also has a lot of beautiful coastal scenery. The north has various extraordinary coastal terrains in the northeast corner and the Yilan Coast National Scenic Area, the North Coast, and the Guanyin Mountain National Scenic Area. The deep and vast blue sky are the characteristics of this lot.

沿途還能看見風光明媚的東部海岸及花東縱谷等奇景，其景色令人讚嘆與驚喜。一路往南，可達陽光四溢且具南國風味的大鵬灣國家風景區，順著山勢一路還可以逛一下充滿原住民風情的茂林國家風景區，一探臺灣蝴蝶世界、魯凱石屋及各色自然美景。

Along the way, you can also see the wonderful scenery of the eastern coast and Huadong Rift Valley, which is amazing and surprising. All the way to the south, you can reach the Dapeng Bay National Scenic Area full of sunshine and southern flavors. You can also visit the Maolin National Scenic Area, which features aboriginal styles along the mountain and explore the world of butterflies, Lukai Stone House, and various natural sceneries.

之所以臺灣的地形會如此構造多變，主要還是因為臺灣位於歐亞板塊與菲律賓海板塊碰撞的交界帶，雖說位處這樣的地帶容易會有地殼不穩定，且地震十分頻繁的問題，但同時也因臺灣位處斷層地帶而擁有眾多的奇特景點，吸引了許多中外遊客前來觀光。

The reason why Taiwan's terrain is so structurally variable is mainly that Taiwan is located at the junction of the collision between the Eurasian Plate and the Philippine Sea plate. Although such a zone is prone to crustal instability and frequent earthquakes, at the same time, because of Taiwan's location in the fault zone, it has many unique attractions, which attract many Chinese and foreign tourists.

而臺灣的氣候構成繁複，北回歸線以北為副熱帶季風氣候，以南為熱帶季風氣候，雖為亞熱帶島嶼，大多數時候平地的氣候溫暖宜人，5 月到 9 月是臺灣的夏季，**每日氣溫經常可達 27 到 35 度**，而夏季長、冬季相對短，冬季受冷空氣影響，相比華南沿海地區顯得更為暖和，但偶而仍會發生低於 10 度的寒潮，且經常冬季降雨，**1 月平均氣溫介於 15~21 度之間**，但由於山脈極高，因此臺灣山區則廣布溫帶植物，冬季北方的雪山山脈甚至會年年降雪。

The climate of Taiwan is complex. The north of the Tropic of Cancer is the subtropical monsoon climate, and the south is the tropical monsoon climate. Although it is a subtropical island, the climate on the flat land is warm and pleasant most of the time. May to September is the summer of Taiwan. **The daily temperature often reaches 27 to 35 degrees Celsius**. The summer is long, while the winter is relatively short. The winter is affected by cold air, which is warmer than the coastal areas of southern China, but occasionally cold waves below 10 degrees will still occur, and frequent winter rainfall. **In January, the average temperature is between 15 and 21 degrees Celsius**, but due to the extremely high mountain range, temperate plants are widespread in the mountainous areas of Taiwan, and it even snows every year in the Snow Mountain range.

在天氣方面，臺灣因為位於歐亞大陸與太平洋的交界帶，因近海陸交界，冷暖洋流（中國沿岸流與黑潮）也在鄰近海域交會，氣候上深受海陸性質差異的影響，也使臺灣經常發生降雨的現象。

In terms of weather, Taiwan is located at the junction of the Eurasian continent and the Pacific Ocean, and because of the offshore land border, the cold and warm ocean currents (Chinese coastal currents and Kuroshio currents) also meet in the adjacent sea area, bringing rainfall in the region.

此外，由於臺灣冬夏季季風會在帶來豐沛的降水，使得臺灣較同緯度的其他國家溼潤，**較不會有空氣乾澀的問題**，在溫度方面，臺灣夏季由於受太平洋高壓影響，氣候較為炎熱，而冬季期間則會因極地冷氣團影響，往往帶來寒冷氣流，但多數情況下不至於寒冷到會出現下雪降霜的現象，雖說臺灣各地因地形與季風影響導致溫差顯著，但由於**臺灣日夜溫差較小**，因此較不會有許多國家早上穿薄紗、晚上穿棉襖的現象。

Moreover, Taiwan’s winter and summer monsoons bring abundant precipitation, making Taiwan more humid than other countries at the same latitude, and **less likely to have dry air**. In terms of temperature, Taiwan’s summer is affected by the Pacific high pressure, and the climate is hotter. During the winter, polar air masses often bring cold air currents, but in most cases, it is not cold enough to cause snow and frost. Although the temperature difference across Taiwan is significant due to the influence of terrain and monsoon, **the temperature difference between day and night in Taiwan is relatively small**, so it is less likely to see the situation of wearing light clothing in the morning and cotton-padded jackets at night like in many countries.

就是因為臺灣深具多樣的地形及特殊的地理位置，使得臺灣的自然環境十分多樣而複雜，高聳的山脈搭配變化多端的海岸景觀，加上冬夏季風的影響，共同交織成豐美多樣的地球之島，而要在臺灣觀賞上述這些地理特徵及奇景，只需要花你在短短幾天的時間便可悉數遊歷。

Because of Taiwan's diverse terrains and unique geographical location, Taiwan's natural environment is very varied and complex. The towering mountains and the changing coastal landscape, combined with the winter and summer monsoon's influence, are interwoven into this island of abundance and diversity. It will only take you a few days of travel to see these geographical features and wonders in Taiwan.

美食天堂 Food Paradis

這個地方有著各國各地的美食選擇

This place provides culinary options from all over the world.

由於臺灣擁有多元的文化及**多次被異國殖民的歷史**，受到長期異國文化的薰陶，在美食的選擇中也顯得比其他國家還要多元，不僅融合閩南、潮州、客家、日本、韓國的飲食文化，甚至融合了歐美文化的飲食特徵，更創造了許多臺灣在地獨有的美食小吃，而最具代表性且廣為國際的想必就是**珍珠奶茶、臭豆腐與皮蛋**了吧！

Due to Taiwan's diverse culture and **the history of being colonized by foreign countries many times,** it has been influenced by foreign cultures for a long time. It also appears to be more diverse in food choices than in other countries. It not only integrates the diets of southern Fujian, Chaozhou,

Hakka, Japan, and South Korea cultures, but created the fusion of the dietary characteristics of European and American culture, and even created many unique food snacks. The most representative and internationally known are **pearl milk tea, stinky tofu, and preserved eggs!**

珍珠奶茶（Bubble tea, Pearl milk tea）是臺灣飲品界**最具國際知名的代表美食**，又稱粉圓奶茶（Tapioca (ball) tea）、波霸奶茶（Boba/Poba milk tea），是 1980 年代起源於臺灣的茶類飲料，為臺灣泡沫紅茶與粉圓茶飲文化中的分支，製作的方法是將粉圓加入奶茶中，另有「珍珠紅（綠）茶」、「珍珠奶綠」等變種，濃郁的奶茶香搭配 Q 彈軟嫩的粉圓，解渴又有嚼勁，口感特殊且讓人欲罷不能，所以廣受世界各地的美食愛好者歡迎及回響，也成為了臺灣最具代表性的飲食。

Bubble tea, or pearl milk tea, is the most famous beverage in Taiwan beverage industry. Also known as Tapioca (ball) tea, Boba/Poba milk tea originated in the 1980s from Taiwan's tea beverages as a branch of the Taiwanese bubble black tea and tapioca ball tea-drinking culture. The method of making it is to add the tapioca balls into the milk tea, and there are other variants such as "pearl black (green) tea" and "pearl milk green". The rich flavor of milk tea with the soft and tender round shape chewy tapioca balls satisfy people's thirst and make one savor on its texture. It has an exceptional taste and makes people simply can't stop wanting to take another sip. Therefore, it is widely welcomed and echoed by food lovers worldwide, and it has become the most representative drink in Taiwan.

關於臺灣珍珠奶茶的起源其實頗有爭議，有兩家臺灣茶飲業者宣稱自己是發明者，一家是源自臺中的春水堂，另一家則是源自臺南的翰林茶館，然而不管到底是誰先發明的，因為這兩家茶飲店皆未對珍珠奶茶申請專利或商標，故才有機會使得珍珠奶茶能被廣為流傳，成為臺灣最具代表性的國民飲品。

The origin of Taiwanese bubble milk tea is quite controversial. Two Taiwanese tea drink stores claim to be the inventor, one is from Chun Shui Tang in Taichung, and the other is from Hanlin Teahouse in Tainan. However, no matter who invented it, because neither of the two tea shops has applied for a patent or trademark for pearl milk tea, pearl milk tea became widely circulated as the most representative national drink in Taiwan.

而臭豆腐跟鐵蛋則是讓多數歐美人士**聞風喪膽**的「極品」美食，之所以這兩道美食會成為國際代表的臺灣美食，那是因為它們那**妙不可聞的味道及邪惡的外觀**導致，偏偏多數臺灣人又喜歡給歐美朋友嘗試這兩種食物，這也因多數未嘗試過這兩種食物的歐美人士會對其味道與外觀充滿恐懼，某些臺灣人這樣的反應很是逗趣。

The stinky tofu and iron eggs are the "gourmet" food that makes most Europeans and Americans **frightened**. These two foods became the international representative of Taiwanese food because of their **intriguing smell and evil appearance**.

However, most Taiwanese like to let their foreign friends try these two foods because most Europeans and Americans who have not tried these two foods are full of fear of their taste and appearance, and some Taiwanese people find such reactions interesting.

但事實上這兩種食物並不如它們的味道與外觀一樣令人害怕，甚至還令人超乎想像的好吃，以下我就來說明它們具體會好吃的原因。

But in fact, these two foods are not as frightening as their smell and appearance and are even more delicious than expected. Allow me to illustrate how delicious they are.

臭豆腐，源自於中國長沙、南京等地，**由豆腐發酵製作而成**，最早傳說發明者是由一個中國清朝的落榜考生在無意間發明而成。雖說大多數臭豆腐都奇臭無比，但卻又都非常好吃，其反差令眾多饕客感到神奇。

Stinky tofu originated from Changsha, Nanjing, and other

places in China is **made from fermented tofu**. According to legend, the inventor was a candidate who failed the exam in the Qing Dynasty in China. Although most stinky tofu is exceptionally stinky, they are very delicious, a contrast that amazed many gluttons.

臭豆腐的種類非常多種，在臺灣最常見兩種分別為**麻辣臭臭鍋**跟**油炸臭豆腐**，麻辣臭臭鍋的煮法一般是以高湯加入少許配料為湯底，之後放入生的臭豆腐乾並注入高湯及加入其他如辣椒、蔥、香菜、醬油等佐料並搭配蔬菜、肉類燉煮而成，非常適合在臺灣冬天的時候食用，其**辣味及臭味後勁無窮**，令人食指大動。

There are many types of stinky tofu, and the two most common in Taiwan are **spicy stinky pot and deep-fried stinky tofu**. Spicy stinky pot is usually made by adding a few ingredients to the soup stock. Then adding dried raw stinky tofu and infused with broth and other condiments such as chili, onion, coriander, soy sauce, etc. Then it is stewed with vegetables and meat, very suitable for winter in Taiwan. **Its spicy taste and odor are endless**, which makes people feel mouthwatering.

麻辣臭臭鍋除了那些早已習慣此等美食的饕客與臺灣本島在地人外，大多數歐美人士皆不敢食用，如果你是勇於挑戰各國料理的美食家，剛好你又喜歡吃辣，那此等美食你絕對不可錯過，因為他將讓你畢生難忘！

In addition to those gluttons and locals who are already accustomed to this food, most Europeans and Americans dare not try it. If you are a foodie who dares to challenge foreign cuisines and happens to like spicy food, you must not miss this dish, because it will be unforgettable all your life!

而油炸臭豆腐則是大**多歐美人士都比較能接受**的臭豆腐了，油炸臭豆腐的製作方式非常簡單，首先料理人會先將臭豆腐丟至油鍋，待炸到外皮酥脆後撈起來朝對角切成四塊再回鍋繼續炸，直到豆腐看起來呈現金黃色後再撈起瀝乾油後裝盤或裝袋。通常在油炸臭豆腐裝盤裝袋的同時，料理人也會將臺灣獨有的「台式」泡菜加入其中，其**酥脆又爽口的特殊口感**令人欲罷不能。身為臺灣土生土長的本地人，我也比較能接受這個版本的臭豆腐，只要你能克服嗅覺的恐懼，那這道料理絕對好吃到你想一吃再吃。

The fried stinky tofu is **more acceptable to most people in Europe and the United States**. The method of making fried stinky tofu is straightforward. First, the cook will throw the stinky tofu into the oil pan, and then fry it until the crust is crispy. Cut it into four pieces diagonally and return to the pan to continue frying until the tofu looks golden brown. Then remove the drained oil and put it in a plate or bag. Usually, while putting the stinky tofu in a plate or bag, the cook will also add Taiwan's unique "tabletop" kimchi. **The special crispy and refreshing taste are finger-licking**. As a native of Taiwan, I also find this version of stinky tofu more acceptable. As long as you can overcome the fear of its smell, this dish is absolutely delicious and you will want to eat it again and again.

再來就是所有歐美人士都無法接受的皮蛋了，相傳皮蛋曾被 CNN 美國有線電視新聞網票選為「全球最噁食物」，由於其黑色的外表常讓不少人誤以為是因儲存過久、重金屬殘留，故被戲稱為**惡魔的蛋**，皮蛋在英文翻譯中也被翻譯成「百年蛋」或「千年蛋」。

Then there is the preserved egg, which is unacceptable to all Europeans and Americans. It is said that preserved egg was once voted as the "world's worst food" by the CNN due to its black appearance, which many people often mistake for storage for too long, or heavy metal residues, so it is dubbed as **the devil's egg**. The preserved egg is also translated as a "hundred-year egg" or "millennium egg" in the English translation.

另外在 2019 年，義大利警方查扣當地華人店鋪 800 顆皮蛋與鹹鴨蛋，並將其形容為這是「不適合人類食用」的食物，可見歐美人士對皮蛋的恐懼有多麼的嚴重。

In 2019, the Italian police seized 800 preserved eggs and salted duck eggs from local Chinese shops and described them as "unsuitable for human consumption." This shows how severely the European and American people fear preserved eggs.

假若你是對臺灣相對不了解的人，又或是三餐都需要搭配皮蛋的人，你肯定會認為我對皮蛋的解說過度加油添醋，但事實上這就是多數稍加了解臺灣的歐美人士對皮蛋的看法。

If you are a person who doesn't know much about Taiwan or someone who needs to have preserved eggs in all three meals, you will definitely think that my explanation of preserved eggs is too exaggerating. Still, as a matter of fact, this is the view of the majority of Europeans and Americans who know a little bit about Taiwan have on preserved eggs.

其實，皮蛋是**以鴨蛋或雞蛋為製作原料的加工食品**，較古老的做法是用輕鹼的混合石灰泥和米糠包裹在鴨蛋外面放在陰涼處三個月以上，再儲存一段時間後蛋的內部便會產生變化，蛋清凝結為膠凍狀、變成半透明黑色，上面有許多淡黃色花紋，極似松樹針狀葉，故又有雅稱松花蛋。

Preserved eggs are **processed foods made from duck eggs or eggs.** The conventional method uses light alkali mixed lime mud and rice bran to wrap the duck eggs outside and put them in a cool place for more than three months. After some storage time, the interior of the egg will change, and the egg white will condense into a jelly shape and become translucent black. There are many light yellow patterns on it, which are very similar to pine needle shaped leaves, given its name pine flower eggs.

由於皮蛋醃製過程中使蛋白質及脂質被分解，因此皮蛋**比一般的雞蛋更容易消化**吸收，且膽固醇含量也變得比蛋還要低。在臺灣，多數感冒發燒的在地人為了減緩感冒進食的不舒適感，多數會選擇食用加入皮蛋與瘦肉的粥來補充營養，至於皮蛋的口感如何，我認為最負責任且最貼切的說法就是就是比較固體的半熟蛋或溫泉蛋，基本上只要不要對它的外觀投射以太多的想像，他就是一個日常可以被接受的主食配料，而且我個人認為其實它比全熟水煮蛋還好吃。

As preserved eggs are decomposed during the curing process of proteins and lipids, preserved eggs are easier to digest and absorb than ordinary eggs. The cholesterol level also becomes lower than the eggs. In Taiwan, many local people who catch a cold and fever choose to eat porridge with preserved eggs and lean meat to supplement nutrition to alleviate the uncomfortable feeling of eating. As for the taste, I think the most responsible and accurate statement is to compare it to solid half-boiled eggs or hot spring eggs. As long as you don't project too much on its appearance, it is a staple ingredient that can be accepted daily, and I personally think it tastes better than fully cooked hard-boiled eggs.

最後再分享一個歐美人士大多不了解的臺灣美食文化，那就是臺灣的早餐店文化，臺灣的早餐店估計是**臺灣展店比例最高的一個產業**了（甚至是媲美臺灣便利商店的數量），基本上每個臺灣人在清晨起床洗漱後的第一件事便是走到附近的早餐店享用早餐。

Finally, I will share a Taiwanese food culture that most Europeans and Americans do not understand: the breakfast store culture in Taiwan. The breakfast stores in Taiwan are estimated to be the industry with **the highest number of stores** (even compared to Taiwanese convenience stores). Generally, the first thing that every Taiwanese do after getting up for wash in the morning is to go to a nearby breakfast store for breakfast.

大多早餐店中除了有中式的豆漿、蛋餅、油條，還有較西式的鬆餅、德式香腸、漢堡、三明治等，非常方便。而之中最受歐美人士歡迎且不多歐美人士知道的美食無遺就是臺灣的「蛋餅」與「米漿」了。

Other than the Chinese-style soybean milk, Chinese omelet with egg and pancakes, most breakfast stores also serve the more Western-style muffins, German sausages, burgers, sandwiches, etc. which is very convenient. Among the most popular foods among Europeans and Americans that not many Europeans and Americans know about are Taiwan's "Chinese omelet with egg " and "brown rice milk."

蛋餅是一種將雞蛋加入麵粉、鹽、蔥或韭菜煎成餅狀，再加上玉米、培根、火腿、起司、蔬菜等佐料，並在煎熟後捲起來的美食，我個人**私心認為是世界上最美味的早餐**，我每天早上都會吃。
Chinese omelet with egg is a dish made by adding eggs into the flour, salt, green onions or leeks, putting in corn, bacon, ham, cheese, vegetables, and other condiments, and rolling it up for eating after frying. I **personally think that it is the most delicious breakfast** in the world. I have it every morning.

另外就是米漿了，它一種用米製成的飲品，通常能接受奶茶的人都能接受這種中式飲料，若說豆漿是中式的牛奶，那我私心認為**米漿就是中式的奶茶**，而且顏色同樣也都非常像，據身邊歐美人士的食用心得表示，這是一杯非常健康的「花生醬」飲料，喝起來有花生醬奶昔的即視感。

Next is brown rice milk. It is a drink made of rice. Anyone who can accept milk tea can take this Chinese drink. If soybean milk is Chinese milk, I think that **brown rice milk is like Chinese milk tea**, and even the color is very similar. According to the experience of people in Europe and America, this is a very healthy "peanut butter" drink, and it tastes like peanut butter milkshake.

若改日有機會來臺灣觀光，還請你早起的時候務必去早餐店點一份蛋餅與一杯米漿，相信你肯定愛上！

If you have the opportunity to visit Taiwan in the future, please order a Chinese omelet with an egg and a cup of brown rice milk at the breakfast store when you get up early. I believe you will love it!

對了！要是你某天來臺灣旅遊，中午的時候千萬不要忘記去附近的店家點一碗牛肉麵或滷肉飯，這個是臺灣的道地美食，若不習慣筷子的人也可以請店家附湯匙食用。

Oh, and if you travel to Taiwan one day, don't forget to order a bowl of beef noodles or braised pork rice at a nearby store at noon. This is authentic Taiwanese food. People who are not used to using chopsticks can also ask the store for a spoon.

晚上的時候我則建議你們可以去臺灣的各大夜市，雖然人很多，但夜市是最快能讓了解臺灣美食風貌的地方（而且臺灣人自己也愛逛，因為夜市裡的東西大多都很便宜），如果你是第一次來臺灣那你就一定要去，它可以快速幫助你了解臺灣。

In the evening, I would suggest that you can go to major night markets in Taiwan. It might be crowded, but the night market is the fastest place to learn about Taiwan's culinary culture (and Taiwanese love to shop there because most of the things in the night market are cheap.), if you are visiting Taiwan for the first time, you must go there, it can help you understand Taiwan quickly.

最後，只要你按照這個行程走訪吃食，你身邊的旅伴肯定會覺得你是一名專業的臺灣美食家與臺灣通，瞬間對你內心的評價加分。

Finally, as long as you visit and eat according to this guide, your travel companions will definitely think that you are a professional Taiwanese foodie who knows Taiwan well and instantly feel impressed.

傳送之門 Portal

這個地方擁有非常方便快速的交通

This place has a very convenient and rapid transportation.

臺灣由於地形因素，東西部交通被中央山脈阻擋，南北部交通由河流所切斷，因此早期臺灣交通極度依賴海運，四千多年前臺灣的史前人類就已經是了不起的航海家，曾坐著小舟把花蓮生產的玉器帶到東南亞各國交易，航路最遠航行到距離臺灣三千多公里的泰國南部的 Khao Sam Kaeo 遺址。

Due to geological factors in Taiwan, the east-west traffic is blocked by the Central Mountain Range, and the north-south traffic cut off by rivers. Therefore, in the early stage, Taiwan's traffic was extremely dependent on sea transportation. More than 4,000 years ago, Taiwan's prehistoric humans were already great navigators, navigating a small boat trading the jade mined in Hualien to Southeast Asian countries. The route sailed the farthest to the Khao Sam Kaeo site in southern Thailand, more than 3,000 kilometers from Taiwan.

十八世紀，隨著漢人移民來台，臺灣南北部常常需要乘船至中國大陸轉乘，直至清朝治理臺灣的末期時間當局才開始大規模整理南北向的陸上交通，至於東西部的連結則分別開闢淡蘭古道、八通關古道等橫越雪山山脈、中央山脈的山間小徑，做為東西部往來的捷徑，值十九世紀後臺灣巡撫劉銘傳更計畫興建臺灣鐵路，從基隆至抵臺南，但後續官員為減輕財政負擔，雖然這條鐵路已測量至大甲溪，卻僅完成基隆至臺北、臺北至新竹兩條路線，但已領先當時中國其他地區的鐵路建設。

In the 18th century, as the Han people immigrate to Taiwan, people in the north and south of Taiwan often needed to take a boat to mainland China for transfers. It was not until the last period of the Qing Dynasty's administration of Taiwan that the authorities began to organize large-scale north-south land traffic. Opening trails across the Xueshan Mountains and the Central Mountains, such as the Danlan Ancient Road and the Batongguan Ancient Road, as a shortcut to the east and west. Taiwan's governor Liu Mingchuan planned to build a Taiwan railway from Keelung to Tainan after the 19th century. However, to reduce the financial burden, the officials after only completed the two routes from Keelung to Taipei and Taipei to Hsinchu, despite this railway has been measured to Dajiaxi. However, it was still ahead of the railway construction in other parts of China at that time.

在日本取得臺灣主權後，臺灣的交通建設網才正式被落實，不但西部鐵路由新竹延伸至屏東縣枋寮，東部的花蓮、臺東之間，也建有窄軌鐵路，而在整個西部平原，糖業、鹽業等專用輕便鐵路更是密布。至於空中交通的部分也是奠定於此時期，但多以軍事機場為主。

It was only after Japan gained sovereignty of Taiwan that Taiwan's transportation construction network was officially implemented. Not only did the Western Railway extend from Hsinchu to Fangliao in Pingtung County, but also the narrow-gauge railway between Hualien and Taitung in the east. Besides, special light railways for industrial use, such as the sugar and salt industries, are densely covered. Air traffic was also established in this period, but mainly military airports.

後來在中華民國政府遷臺時，面對海峽兩岸關係情勢的危機，早期的交通建設則以軍事防衛為主，而後來的高速公路與高速鐵路則是以在近數十年的十大建設計劃中一一完工，再加上國內航空路網的建構，以及各大城市軌道交通系統、南北高速鐵路的興築，今日臺灣交通的面貌才逐漸完成。

Later, when the government of the Republic of China relocated to Taiwan, facing the crisis of cross-strait relations, the early transportation infrastructure was designed for the primary purpose of military defense. The highways and high-speed railways built after followed the top ten construction plans in recent decades. Coupled with the construction of the domestic aviation road network, the construction of the rail transit system in major cities, and the construction of the North-South high-speed railway, the appearance of Taiwan's transportation is gradually completed today.

前幾個小節有提到，臺灣是一個四面環海且總面積約為 36,000 平方公里的一個小島國。由於其國土面積較小，所以也相對容易**一覽無遺全島風光**，且現今因交通選擇繁多，**不必太過擔心會有迷路或在荒郊野外與人群失聯**的問題，更不必擔心沒有交通工具可以搭乘。

As mentioned in the previous sections, Taiwan is a small island country surrounded by the sea and covering a total area of approximately 36,000 square kilometers. Due to its small land area, it is **relatively easy to see the island’s beautiful landscapes**. Due to the many transportation options today, there is **no need to worry too much about getting lost or losing contact with people in the wilderness.**

此外，臺灣的鐵路及捷運建設也相當完善，除了高速鐵路外，在北區也能選擇以捷運或客運的方式交通，另外臺灣也有很多的小黃（由於臺灣的計程車多會漆成黃色，故有小黃這個暱稱），如果你搭不習慣計程車或怕計程車坐地起價你也可以選擇 Uber，臺灣有支援 Uber 的系統（雖然臺灣的計程車完全不會有這個問題就是，而且臺灣大多計程車司機還會穿襯衫打領帶，並提供免費的當地旅遊嚮導資訊，是觀光旅客 CP 值非常高的選項）。

In addition, Taiwan's railway and MRT systems are also quite complete. Other than high-speed railways, MRT or intercity buses can also be chosen in the North District. Besides, Taiwan also has many Xiao Huang (because Taiwan's taxis are mostly painted yellow, so there is the nickname Xiao Huang, meaning Little Yellow). If you are not used to taking taxis or are afraid that the taxi fares will be outrageous, you can also choose Uber.

Taiwan has a system that supports Uber (although Taiwan's taxis will not have this problem, and most taxi drivers in Taiwan wear a shirt and tie and provide free local travel guide information, which is a very high-value option for tourists.)

註：如果你在臺灣想要享受美食，卻又不想出飯店，這時你可以選擇 food panda 或 uber eat 這兩個外送平台 APP，裡面有眾多美食選擇任君挑選。

Note: If you want to enjoy the food in Taiwan, but don't want to go out of the hotel, you may choose to order from either of the two food delivery platform apps, Food Panda or Uber Eat, which provides a wide range of cuisine options.

在臺灣，若你想要前往綠島、蘭嶼等離島，你可以選擇飛機或快艇，但如果你想體驗海上度假時光，你可以選擇購買遊艇的旅遊行程，運氣好的話還能在海上度假期間看到海豚或鯨魚。

In Taiwan, if you want to go to the outlying islands such as Green Island and Orchid Island, you can choose to take the airplane or motorboat, but if you want to experience sea vacation time, a yacht tour package comes highly recommended. If you are lucky, you might even see dolphins or whales.

而公路系統的部分則遍及臺灣島及澎湖群島各鄉鎮，若是你想租賃汽車進行一趟在台公路旅行的話也是非常方便，而如果你只是想租賃摩托車，也可以下載 **WeMo、GoShare、iRent** 等共享機車 APP，它不僅可以幫你自動定位哪個地方有租賃機車，還有許多划算的租賃方案，讓你可以以最小成本玩遍臺灣各地。

The highway system covers all towns in Taiwan and the Penghu Islands. It is also very convenient if you want to rent a car for a road trip in Taiwan. If you want to rent a motorcycle, you can also download share vehicle apps such as **WeMo, GoShare, iRent**, and more, that not only can help you automatically locate a rental locomotive, but also provide many cost-effective rental packages, enabling you to travel all over Taiwan at minimum cost.

最後，雖說臺灣是一個沒這麼大的島國，但為了方便在地公民，我們的政府也落實了許多交通建設及扶植民間各個交通產業，這不僅讓一般民眾的生活更加便利（**搭乘高速鐵路從最北到最南只需兩三個小時**），也降低了觀光客來此處觀光的門檻。若你剛來到臺灣，且不介意行程緊湊的話，那你可以考慮七天遊臺灣的行程，你能在這段期間體驗到非常多新奇好玩的事物。

Finally, although Taiwan is not a very big island country, our government has implemented many transportation infrastructures and support for the various private transportation sector for the benefit of local citizens. It makes the lives of ordinary people more convenient **(it takes only 2-3 hours to travel from the northernmost to the southernmost by the high-speed railway)** and lowers the threshold for tourists to come here for sightseeing. If you have just arrived in Taiwan and don't mind the tight schedule, you can consider a seven-day trip traveling the entire Taiwan, where you can experience a lot of new and exciting things.

還有！如果你在臺灣遊玩時找不到路，除了使用 Google map 之外，你也可以詢問路上的行人，就算這些人可能不懂你的語言，但他們也會盡可能地幫助你找到你想要去的位置。

Moreover, if you can’t find your way while visiting Taiwan, you can also ask the pedestrians on the road besides using Google Maps. Even if these people may not understand your language, they will try their best to help you find the direction of where you want to go.

炎黃古跡 Chinese Cultural Heritage

這個地方保存著昔日的文明與禮儀

This place preserves past culture and etiquette.

在前面眾多小節提到，臺灣是一個多元文化的國家，其原因不光是因為有被多國殖民及傳教的歷史經驗，更因臺灣在地民眾從他國帶回來的技術和知識影響，因此在臺灣你能看到許多各國文化結合的產物，甚至就連過去的歷史建築也充滿著東西文化融合的味道。

As mentioned in the many previous sections, Taiwan is a country of multiculturalism. The reason is not only because of the historical experience of being colonized and preached by many countries but also because of the influence of technology and knowledge brought back from other countries by the people of Taiwan. Therefore, in Taiwan, you can see the many things that are a combination or integration of various cultures, even the historical buildings feature a fusion of oriental and western culture.

若要淺談臺灣的多元文化，那就得先從臺灣的原民文化及殖民歷史說起，臺灣在過**去的時代曾歷經過多國文化的政權交替**，從最早期的南島文化、古閩粵文化，地理大發現後開始的荷蘭、葡萄牙、西班牙殖民者帶來的早期西方文化，明鄭時期以後東南沿海漢族開始大規模開墾帶來的閩南文化、客家文化及引進儒家、道家和佛教等宗教思想與東方禮儀，再到後來混合日治殖民的日本文化影響，讓臺灣不僅擁有健全的文化底蘊，更賦予了臺灣當地人民傳承多國的東西方禮儀，同時也讓**臺灣人民擁有樂於佈施及尊師重道的崇高道德素養**。

If we are to discuss Taiwan's multiculturalism briefly, we will have to start with Taiwan's aboriginal culture and colonial history. In the past, **Taiwan has gone through the regimes of many different cultures;** Starting from the earliest Austronesian culture and ancient Fujian and Guangdong culture to the early Western culture brought by the Dutch, Portuguese, and Spanish colonists after the Age of Discovery, to the southern Fujian culture, Hakka culture. Then philosophical thoughts and oriental etiquettes of Confucianism, Taoism, and Buddhism were brought by the Han people's large-scale reclamation on the southeast coast after the Ming and Zheng period, and later the Japanese cultural influence of Japanese colonization. Taiwan not only has a complete cultural heritage but endowed with the traditions and etiquette of both the East and the West, which at the same time grant the people of Taiwan **the noble moral qualities of being willing to give as well as respecting and honoring elderlies and teachers.**

20 世紀，臺灣受戰後美國文化影響、本地與臺灣原住民的文化復興，同時又經歷印尼，越南等東協國家大量移民，對臺灣的語言及文化造成了多元豐富的碰撞，也因此臺灣的文化具有**融合傳統與現代、東方與西方**等共同面向，以臺灣為主體的文化範疇逐漸在世界確立。

In the 20th century, Taiwan was influenced by the post-war American culture, the cultural revival of local and Taiwanese aborigines, while at the same time experienced a massive influx of immigrants from Indonesia, Vietnam and other ASEAN countries. It leads to a diverse and vibrant collision with Taiwan's language and culture. Subsequently, Taiwan's culture orients toward **an integration of the tradition and modernity, the East and the West**, and gradually transformed into its unique characters and established its role in the world.

從臺灣使用的傳統面向看來，臺灣使用的漢字是**繁體字**，又稱為正體字，同時又為中國文化的正統漢字。在中華人民共和國政府進行簡化前並沒有繁體字一說，只有正體字與俗體字之分，而簡體字支持者認為，文字變革是自然的事，用正體字來稱呼傳統漢字有暗示簡體字為「歪體」之嫌。

From the perspective of traditional Chinese characters used in Taiwan, the Chinese characters used in Taiwan are **traditional characters**, also known as orthodox characters, and at the same time are the orthodox Chinese characters of Chinese culture. Before the government of the People's Republic of

China simplified Chinese characters, there was no such thing as traditional characters, only a distinction between regular and vulgar characters. Supporters of simplified characters believe that characters' change is a natural evolution; calling traditional Chinese characters orthodox characters implies that simplified characters are "distorted".

在歷經中國多代歷史的演變，對於傳統漢字與簡化字的爭議已久，曾經在中華文化圈廣泛使用的傳統正體漢字現在**銳減為簡體字用戶的三十三分之一**，這更顯得臺灣傳統文化的珍貴性及彰顯臺灣保存珍貴文化的能力。

After many generations of history in China, there has been a long-standing dispute over traditional Chinese characters and simplified characters. The traditional Chinese characters that were once widely used in the Chinese cultural circle have now been **drastically reduced to one thirty-third of people who use simplified characters.** It further shows the preciousness of the traditional culture preserved by Taiwan and also Taiwan' s ability to protect precious culture.

從臺灣現代的文化發展面向敘述，前提說道，20 世紀臺灣受戰後美國文化影響，天主教與基督新教在臺灣地方宗教文化中的佔據著非常重要的角色，如台語詩歌的改編，偏遠地區地方教堂的貢獻等，此外就是在教育方面，鑑於歐美現代教育的精神在臺灣教育界中往往被引為典範，近年來臺灣的教育改革政策也開始效仿歐美教育的精神。

From the narrative of Taiwan's modern cultural development, the premise is that in the 20th century, Taiwan was influenced by post-war American culture. Catholicism and Protestantism played a significant role in Taiwan's local religious customs, such as adapting Taiwanese poetry and the church's contributions in remote areas, etc. Moreover, in the aspect of education, since the spirit of modern European and American education is often taken as a model in Taiwan's education circles, in recent years, Taiwan's education reform policies have begun to emulate the spirit of European and American education.

至於其他領域現代化的部分，鑑於歐美文化的影視薰陶，在很多亞洲地區國家中都逐漸開始能看到文化西化的影子，就例如好萊塢為代表的美國電影文化等。而傳承歐美的現代建築思想也逐漸被臺灣的建築設計師導入臺灣，如玻璃帷幕的摩天大樓，集合式的社區公寓，河濱公園等，也影響了臺灣的建築文化發展走向，其西方現代化的建築特色，更能彰顯出臺灣**傳統文化建築與創新文化交織碰撞**的特殊韻味。

As for the modernization of other fields, given the influence of European and American culture in film and television, many Asian countries are gradually beginning to shadow cultural westernization, such as the American film culture represented by Hollywood. The modern architectural ideas inherited from Europe and the United States are steadily introduced into Taiwan by Taiwanese architects. For example, skyscrapers with glass curtains, collective community apartments, riverside parks, etc., have also affected Taiwan's architectural culture's development trend. The architectural features can further

demonstrate the unique charm of the interweaving and collision of Taiwan's traditional cultural architecture and innovative culture.

此外，再 20 世紀中，中華國民政府遷台期間，為保當時留存的古物不遭受戰爭破壞，故透過海運運送近**五千箱殘留文物**，其中不僅包含各式珍貴藏書及外交文書，更包含宋、元、明、清中國四朝的宮廷收藏，也為臺灣正統的中國歷史文化傳承奠定了紮實的根基。

In addition, during the relocation of the Chinese Nationalist Government to Taiwan in the middle of the 20th century, to protect the antiquities preserved at that time from being damaged by war, nearly **5,000 boxes of cultural relics** were transported by sea, including not only various precious collections and diplomatic documents, but also the imperial court collections of the four dynasties of China, Song, Yuan, Ming, and Qing, which also laid a solid foundation for Taiwan's heritage of orthodox Chinese history and culture.

最後，若你有機會走訪臺灣，由於臺灣本島的城鎮發展是由**台南、彰化及台北**三處開始，故這三處城市中**留存的古蹟建築眾多**，其中曾為臺灣統治中心的台南和台北兩地的古蹟數量更**超過百處**，如果你想透過旅遊親身體會臺灣的歷史文化底蘊，這三處是你絕對要走訪的城市。

Finally, if you have the opportunity to visit Taiwan, since the development of cities and towns on Taiwan's main island started in **Tainan, Changhua, and Taipei**, **many historical monuments and buildings** remain in these three cities. Among them, Tainan and Taipei were the Taiwanese rule centers with **more than a hundred** historical sites. If you want to experience Taiwan's historical and cultural heritage through tourism, these three are the cities you absolutely must visit.

而在臺灣外島的金門及澎湖的部分，由於這兩地為早期海峽船隻往來的必經之處，故開發的比臺灣本島早，在這你不僅能看到**燈塔及碉堡**等建築，並可以感受到充分的島嶼風情及殖民文化。

In the parts of Kinmen and Penghu on the outer islands of Taiwan, since these two places were necessary routes for ships to pass through the strait in the early years, they were developed earlier than the main island of Taiwan. Here you can see buildings such as **lighthouses and bunkers** and feel the island style and colonial culture.

這些古蹟不僅為臺灣述說了其豐富的殖民歷史，更讓人能深刻體會到當代殖民者在臺灣殖民的心境及當時人民的感受，再加上臺灣健全的都市發展規劃。
These monuments tell Taiwan’s rich colonial history and give people a deep understanding of the mood of colonists in Taiwan and the feelings of the people at that time and Taiwan’s well-rounded urban development plan.

在臺灣，你不僅能感受到東西文化交織合壁的奇特景象，更能直接感受到傳統與現代文化碰撞融合的奇妙體悟，令人賞心悅目、發人省思。

In Taiwan, you can feel the unique characteristics of the interweaving of Eastern and Western cultures and directly contact the wonderful experience of the collision and integration of traditional and modern cultures, which is pleasant and thought-provoking.

護臺灣、助世界

臺灣能幫忙，而且臺灣正在幫忙

Taiwan can help
and Taiwan is helping

第三章
Chapter 3

臺灣能助你
Taiwan Can Help

資源助你 In Resources

或許你們需要更多的資源隔絕病毒

Perhaps you need more resources to block the virus

臺灣總統於 4 月 1 日宣佈，臺灣將「基於人道考量」，捐贈 1000 萬片口罩給全球疫情嚴重國家的醫護人員。

The President of Taiwan announced on April 1 that Taiwan would donate 10 million masks to medical staff in severely affected countries around the world "based on humanitarian considerations."

前面章節多有提到，鑑於臺灣超前部署的政策做得相當成功，在臺灣全體人民努力下，臺灣疫情得到了最好的控制，更透過政府與本地廠商合作、口罩實名制、出入境管制、口罩管制措施、口罩線上訂購等眾多醫療政策實施，讓臺灣不僅從過去的口罩進口國轉變成全球第二大口罩生產國，突破過去產量，單日已經可以**生產出超過一千萬片口罩**，而人口僅有 2300 多萬人的臺灣目前已有充分餘力援助疫情嚴重的國家。

As mentioned in the previous chapters, given that Taiwan's advanced preparation policies have been quite successful, the pandemic has been best controlled through the efforts of all the people in Taiwan. Moreover, through cooperation between the government and local manufacturers, masks rationing, border control, and mask enforcement, many medical policies such as control measures and online mask ordering have transformed Taiwan from a mask importing country in the past to the second-largest mask manufacturer in the world. It has broken past production limits and can already produce **more than 10 million masks in a single day**. Taiwan, which has only 23 million people, now has enough power to assist countries with severe epidemics.

疫情期間，我們捐贈美國 200 萬口罩片、義大利、西班牙、德國、法國、比利時、荷蘭、盧森堡、捷克、波蘭、英國和瑞士等歐洲國家共 700 萬片口罩，以及臺灣邦交國 100 萬片口罩，本次捐贈給 15 個邦交國的口罩也已經分批運送，將陸續運抵各國。

During the pandemic, we donated 2 million masks to the United States, Italy, Spain, Germany, France, Belgium, the Netherlands, Luxembourg, Czech, Poland, the United Kingdom, Switzerland and other European countries with a total of 7 million masks, and 1 million masks to countries with diplomatic relations with Taiwan. The masks donated to 15 countries with diplomatic ties this time have also been shipped in batches and will be shipped to various countries one after another.

面對全球疫情肆虐，我國後續也陸續提出多項人道援助計劃，除前陣子捐贈總數 6 百萬片醫療口罩給北歐、中歐、東歐地區等歐盟會員國外，美洲國家部分我們捐贈口罩給疫情受創嚴重的拉丁美等洲、加勒比海、新南向國家及其他友好國家，另我們也捐贈加拿大政府 40 萬片醫療口罩、安大略省 5 萬片、亞伯達省 2 萬 5 千片、卑詩省、2 萬 5 千片口罩，總計 50 萬片口罩，支援前線醫療人員。

In the face of the raging global pandemic, our country proposed a series of humanitarian assistance programs. In addition to the previous donation of a total of 6 million medical masks to European Union members such as in Northern Europe, Central Europe, and Eastern Europe, in America, we also donated masks to countries that have been severely affected by the pandemic such as in the Latin America, the Caribbean, the New Southbound countries and other friendly countries. We also donated 400,000 medical masks to the Canadian government, 50,000 to Ontario, 25,000 to Alberta, and 25,000 masks to British Columbia, a total of 500,000 masks, to support frontline medical personnel.

而亞洲人道救援計劃的部分，也因臺日雙方每逢天然災害發生時均能相互伸出援手，綜合考量臺日雙方疫情發展及臺灣口罩產能持續提升等因素，我國決定向日本提供 200 萬片口罩協助日方抗疫，強化雙方防疫合作發展，深厚穩固的友誼。

As for the Asian humanitarian aiding plan, because Taiwan and Japan lend a hand to each other whenever natural disasters occur. Considering factors such as the development of the epidemic in Taiwan and Japan and the continuous increase in Taiwan's mask production capacity, our country has decided to provide Japan with 2 million pieces to help Japan fight the epidemic. It will strengthen the cooperation and development of epidemic prevention between the two sides, maintaining a deep and stable friendship.

另由於在義大利境內的天主教教會、文教社福設施、及相關神職等人員受到新冠病毒疫情的嚴重影響，繼日臺灣政府人道援贈 28 萬片口罩給教廷及所屬包括靈醫會在內的天主教團體後，為感念天主教神職人員對臺灣過去在接受傳教期間多次受神職人員的醫療援助，更對臺灣文化普及教育有著不可或缺的貢獻，我國政府決定加贈 20 萬片醫療口罩，以幫助教廷度過難關。

Moreover, because the Catholic Church, cultural, educational, and social welfare facilities, and related priests in Italy have been severely affected by the COVID-19, the Taiwanese government has donated 280,000 masks to the Holy See and its affiliates, including the Camillians. Furthermore, in appreciation of the medical assistance provided by the Catholic clergy to Taiwan in the past during the missionary period, and the indispensable contribution to the popularization of Taiwan's culture and education, the Taiwan government decided to donate an additional 200,000 pieces of medical masks to help the Holy See through the difficulties.

然而，我們深知僅僅捐贈如此數量的醫療資源是遠遠不足以讓世界面對新冠肺炎疫情的持續擴散的，於是我國將在

後續啟動第三波國際人道援助行動，並納入臺灣國人響應「護臺灣，助世界」的自主捐贈行動，捐贈總計 707 萬片醫療口罩，其中包括給美國聯邦政府及疫情嚴峻各州 228 萬片、歐盟及其會員國 130 萬片、我各邦交國 109 萬片，以及新南向相關國家共 180 萬片，另將提供部分非洲及中東國家與協助敘利亞難民的醫護人員共 60 萬片口罩。

However, we are fully aware that just donating such a amount of medical resources is far from enough to allow the world to face the continual spread of the COVID-19. Therefore, Taiwan **will launch a third wave of international humanitarian assistance operations in the follow-up** and include Taiwanese people's response to "Protect Taiwan, Help the World" initiative which donated a total of 7.07 million medical masks, including 2.28 million to the U.S. federal government and states where conditions are severe, 1.3 million to the European Union and its member countries, 1.09 million to countries with diplomatic relations with Taiwan, and provide a total of 1.8 million pieces of masks to countries related to New

Southbound. A total of 600,000 pieces of masks to the medical staff assisting Syrian refugees in some African and Middle Eastern countries.

防疫無國界，面對新冠肺炎疫情各國皆無法獨善其身，我們唯有透過互助互利的合作才能築起堅實的抗疫防線。同時！在國際社會正強化防疫機制的期間，臺灣有意願且也有能力與各國建立防疫合作，並貫徹「**臺灣能幫忙，而且臺灣正在幫忙**」的決心持續以實際行動應證，具體展現臺灣政府與全體 2,300 萬人民的愛心、信心與參與國際事務的誠意與決心。

Epidemic prevention knows no borders. In the face of the coronavirus, no country can stand alone. Only through mutually beneficial cooperation can we build a solid line of defense against the epidemic. Simultaneously! While the international community is strengthening the anti-epidemic mechanism, Taiwan has the willingness and ability to establish cooperation with other countries in pandemic prevention, demonstrate the determination of **"Taiwan can help, and Taiwan is helping"** and proving it with practical actions, concretely showing the love, confidence, sincerity, and dedication of Taiwanese government and the entire 23 million population of Taiwan in participating in international affairs.

技術助你 In Technology

或許你們需要更多的技術制止病毒

Perhaps you need more technology support in stopping the virus.

---

3 月 18 日，我國外交部與美國在台協會同步公開「臺美防疫夥伴關係聯合聲明」，指為共同對抗源自中國武漢的武漢肺炎病毒台美雙方將進一步強化諮商與合作機制。

On March 18, the Ministry of Foreign Affairs of our country and the American Association in Taiwan simultaneously published the "Taiwan-US Joint Statement on a Partnership against Coronavirus," stating that Taiwan and the United States will further strengthen the consultation and cooperation mechanism to jointly combat the Wuhan pneumonia virus originated in Wuhan, China.

其中計劃提到六大抗疫措施，包括快篩檢驗試劑的研發、疫苗的研究與生產、藥品的研究與生產、追蹤接觸者相關技術機制與科技、舉行科學家與專家的聯合會議、防疫醫療用品及裝置的合作與交流。

The plan mentions six primary anti-epidemic measures, including the research and development of rapid screening tests, research, and production of vaccines, research and production of medicines, contact tracing techniques and technology, joint conferences by scientists and experts, as well as cooperation and exchanges of medical supplies and equipment.

除了新藥、快篩方面等六大開發合作之外，為了確保在研發期間防疫物資不致匱乏，美國也已特地為臺灣保留三十萬件防護衣原料，充實臺灣防護物資，讓第一線辛苦的醫護人員可以安心為國際抗疫事業盡心，而在臺灣也將在每週提供十萬片口罩給美國，強化台美抗疫合作。

In addition to new medicines, rapid tests, and the six major development cooperations, in order to ensure that anti-epidemic materials are not scarce during the research and development period, the United States has also specially reserved 300,000 protective clothing materials for Taiwan to enrich Taiwan's protective materials and make sure the frontline medical staff could focus on the international fight against the epidemic, and Taiwan will also provide 100,000 masks to the United States every week to strengthen Taiwan-US cooperation in the fight against the epidemic.

此外，於 3 月 22 日期間，花蓮門諾醫院麻醉科醫師釋出「插管箱」醫療設備設計圖公開無償下載，訊息公開後已有 30 多國開始採用，經美國波士頓醫療中心測試，醫護人員可以透過此設備減少 95%以上的醫療飛沫污染風險。

In addition to new medicines, rapid tests, and the six major development cooperations, to ensure that anti-epidemic materials are not scarce during the research and development period, the United States has also specially reserved 300,000 protective clothing materials for Taiwan to enrich Taiwan's protective materials and make sure the frontline medical staff could focus on the international fight against the epidemic. Taiwan will also provide 100,000 masks to the United States every week to strengthen Taiwan-US cooperation in the fight against the epidemic.

而為什麼臺灣能擁有如此的醫療技術實力與美國進行防疫合作開發呢？
And why can Taiwan have such a medical technology strength to cooperate with the United States in the development of epidemic prevention?

除過去臺灣較常發生傳染病危機外，另也因臺灣醫療就學及從業門檻較高，必須要是臺灣教育體系中**最聰明且最優秀的學生**才能就讀，且醫學系學生必須接受為期 7 年的醫學教育，再經過 4 年住院醫師及專科醫師考試才能成為合格的主治醫師。

In addition to the frequent occurrence of infectious disease in Taiwan in the past, Taiwan's medical education and employment thresholds are relatively high. Only the **brightest and most outstanding** students in Taiwan's education system can enroll in medical school. Moreover, medical students must receive seven years of education, and only after four years of residency and specialist examinations, can you become a qualified attending physician.

平均來說，一名醫學系的學生要成為一個主治醫師必須花費 12 到 13 年的時間。
On average, it takes 12 to 13 years for a medical student to become an attending physician.

另外，臺灣的醫療機構使用的是世界最先進的醫療儀器，例如：電腦斷層掃描器、核磁共振儀及正子攝影技術來作癌症篩檢，冷凍消融、氬氦刀冷凍治療及影像導引放射治療癌症等，也因**臺灣醫師分工專業**，不僅可避免任何個人判斷偏差，更能給予患者及家屬最專業且最簡單易懂的病理及手術方法解釋等，都可以獲得醫師簡單易懂的解釋。

Taiwan's medical institutions use the world's most advanced medical equipment, such as computed tomography, nuclear magnetic resonance, and positron photography for cancer screening, cryoablation, cryotherapy, and image-guided radiotherapy for cancer treatment, etc. Due **to the division of labor between Taiwanese physicians**, they cannot only avoid any personal judgment bias, but they can also provide patients and their families with the most professional and easy-to-understand explanations of pathology and surgical methods.

故此，臺灣甚至獲得了**醫療技術全球第三、亞洲第一**的國際殊榮，同時也因為如此，臺灣不僅擁有充分的醫療資源能協助國際抗疫，更有一群專業且落實「臺灣能幫忙，而且臺灣正在幫忙」決心的醫師團隊，不僅能提供專業的醫療知識協助，更能共享防疫技術，加快國際抗疫事業的發展進程。

Therefore, Taiwan has even won **the third international honor of medical technology in the world and the first in Asia.** At the same time, because of this, Taiwan not only has sufficient medical resources to assist the international fight against the epidemic but also has a group of professionals to implements "Taiwan can help, and Taiwan is helping." This team of determined doctors can provide professional medical knowledge and share anti-epidemic technologies and accelerate international anti-epidemic development.

最後，再經我國政府及民間多年來鍥而不捨的努力，爭取參與世界衛生組織的訴求已經獲得 29 國行政部門、43 個國家或區域的立法部門及數百位各國國會議員及政要的國際支持，這將支持我國的動能不斷累積，並以此證明臺灣堅持「**專業、務實、有貢獻**」的原則是正確的，我國成功防疫及抗疫的「臺灣模式」(Taiwan Model)更獲得國際讚譽，讓國際社會更加正視將臺灣納入WHO的必要性及急迫性，友邦及理念相近國家並以空前強勁的力道支持我國，在此我們臺灣全國 2300 萬人民深受感謝，你們的支持令我們倍受感動，這將是鼓舞我們繼續為國際奉獻的動力。

Finally, after years of persistent efforts by the Taiwanese government and the private sectors, the appeal to participate in the World Health Organization has gained international support from the executive departments of 29 countries, the legislative departments of 43 countries or regions, and hundreds of parliamentarians and dignitaries. It will support Taiwan's continuous accumulation of momentum and prove that Taiwan's insistence on the principle of "**professionalism, pragmatism, and contribution**" is correct. The "Taiwan Model" in epidemic prevention and fight has gained international acclaim, letting the international community see the necessity and urgency of including Taiwan in the WHO. Friends and countries with similar ideas have supported Taiwan with unprecedented strength. Here we, the 23 million people across Taiwan, are deeply grateful to you. Your support has moved us all. It will be the motivation that encourages us to continue to contribute to the world.

也感謝 60 多國媒體的支持，為數共超過 1,800 篇以報導、評論、專欄、投書等方式表達對臺灣的支持，這將是支持臺灣參與國際抗疫事業的強大聲浪。

We also want to appreciate the support of the media from more than 60 countries. More than 1,800 articles have expressed support for Taiwan in the form of reports, comments, columns, and submissions. This will be a loud voice supporting Taiwan's participation in the international anti-epidemic cause.

護臺灣、助世界

臺灣能幫忙，而且臺灣正在幫忙

Taiwan can help
and Taiwan is helping

第四章
Chapter 4

戰疫知識共享
Share Knowledge in fighting the Pandemic

戰術背包 Tactical Backpack
如果你要出門，你得要帶這些東西
If you are going out, you should pack these.

鑑於臺灣過去有豐富的抗疫經驗，且加上本次政府對新冠肺炎的超前部署及臺灣民眾提前獲得中國相關瘟疫傳播的關鍵資訊，非但此次可以避免過去 SARS 必須隔離 15 萬人才能勉強抗疫的慘痛經驗，更讓我國人民毋須擔心因此次疫情與至親家屬愛人天人永隔的命運。

Given that Taiwan has had abundant anti-epidemic experiences in the past, coupled with the government's advanced deployment for the coronavirus and Taiwanese people's access to key information on the spread of China's related plague in advance. It successfully prevented the painful situation of having to quarantine 150,000 people like in SARS to fight the virus barely from happening again and enable our people to be free of the worry about the fate of being separated from their loved ones by this epidemic.

不過，此次我國能有效防疫不光是政府推行的眾多政策所致，更因臺灣有多次面對瘟疫的防疫本人。由於臺灣在抗疫措施實行良善的結果，**<u>臺灣人並未受到疫情強迫停班停課的影響</u>**，也因此臺灣人多數會在出門時會準備自己的防疫「戰術背包」以防未知病毒的侵襲，再此就與你分享臺灣人在外出的情況會攜帶哪些裝備抵抗瘟疫，並會介紹雖只有少數人會攜帶，但非常有用的裝備：

However, my country's effective epidemic prevention this time is due to the numerous policies implemented by the government and because Taiwan has faced plagues many times. Due to the good results of Taiwan's anti-epidemic measures, **<u>Taiwanese have not been affected by the forced suspension of classes and classes due to the epidemic</u>**. Therefore, most Taiwanese will prepare their own anti-epidemic "tactical backpacks" when they go out to prevent the invasion of unknown viruses. I will share with you what equipment Taiwanese will carry to fight the virus when they go out, and introduce the handy equipment that only a few people will carry:

1. 充足的口罩後備資源

Sufficient number of masks

居家旅遊兩相宜，優良的攜帶式抗疫設備。鑑於臺灣過去受日本影響的口罩文化及政府推行的口罩實名制政策，不僅多數人能接受在防疫期間戴上口罩，且能在保證口罩不消耗殆盡的前提下有效使用（在臺灣未有口罩實名制政策前，多數人會因為缺乏口罩儲備而重複使用口罩，且因多數人未能購買到口罩，故在當時不少人暴露在被瘟疫感染的風險中）。

Good for home and travel, excellent portable anti-epidemic equipment. In view of the mask culture in Taiwan that was influenced by Japan in the past and the government's mask rationing system policy, not only can most people accept wearing masks during the epidemic prevention period, but they can also use them effectively while ensuring that masks are not exhausted (Before the policy, most people would reuse masks because of lack of mask reserves, and because most people could not buy masks, many people were exposed to the risk of being infected by the virus at that time).

另外！口罩的種類使用也是一門非常重要的學問，由於臺灣在口罩使用上有多次宣導，故鮮少並有使用無效口罩防疫的事件發生，但鑑於許多國家並未有口罩種類挑選宣導機制，故在這裡稍微解釋一下。

The type and use of masks are also critical. Since Taiwan has repeatedly promoted the use of masks, rarely do cases of using invalid masks to prevent epidemics occur. However, since many countries do not have a mechanism for selecting and promoting mask types, we will briefly explain it.

通常，臺灣人會使用的口罩選擇為 N95 口罩、一般醫用口罩、外科口罩及綁帶式外科口罩，除此之外的口罩都不建議。會使用這些口罩最關鍵的原因是，大多這些口罩都擁有 95%以上的細菌過濾率，並且都可以阻擋 90%5 微米以上的微小因子（N95 口罩能阻擋 3 微米以上的微小因子）。因此，使用這些口罩不光能減少口沫傳染的機率，更能有效降低傳染的可能。

Generally, the masks that Taiwanese will use are N95 masks, general medical masks, surgical masks, and band-type surgical masks. Other masks are not recommended. The most important reason for using these masks is that most of these masks have a bacterial filtration rate of more than 95%, and can block 90% of airborne particles above 5 microns (N95 masks can block airborne particles above 3 microns). Therefore, the use of these masks can reduce the chance of droplet infection and effectively reduce the possibility of infection.

不過，就連在防疫策略實施優秀的臺灣也有少數人會攜帶防毒面具，雖說略顯浮誇，但如果你真的沒有上述口罩資源的話，你可以思考一下你國家中是否有面臨防毒面具缺貨的問題，如果沒有，那你就可以考慮將它放入你的防疫戰術背包。

However, even in Taiwan, where the epidemic prevention strategy is excellent, few people wear gas masks. Although it is a bit exaggerated, if you don't have the mask as mentioned earlier, you can think about if there is a shortage of gas masks in your country. If not, then you may consider putting it in your epidemic prevention tactical backpack.

2. 隨身酒精攜帶瓶

Carry portable disinfection alcohol

在臺灣略顯浮誇的裝備，少數防疫意識較高的臺灣人會隨身攜帶。

會說在臺灣會略顯浮誇的原因是，由於我國在各大公司行號及觀光區域等位置在疫情期間皆有政策要求準備消毒酒精及額溫槍，因此大多臺灣人並不會隨身攜帶，但如果你的國家沒有這項政策，我會建議你隨身攜帶，因為新冠肺炎的傳染途徑有接觸傳染的可能，多一項能消毒的工具更能保障你的生命安全。

A piece of slightly exaggerated equipment in Taiwan, only carried by a small number of Taiwanese with high awareness of epidemic prevention.

It is said to be exaggerating in Taiwan because there is the policy that disinfection alcohol and forehead thermometers are required in major companies and tourist areas during the epidemic period. Therefore, most Taiwanese do not carry it with them. But if your country does not have this policy, I would suggest that you take it with you, because the transmission of coronavirus may be contagious through contact. One more disinfectant tool can better protect your life.

3. 口罩保存攜帶夾

Maskeeper

比上述隨身酒精攜帶瓶更少人會攜帶的防疫設備，但由於攜帶方便，我出門的時候都會帶。

鑑於臺灣有前提多次敘述到的口罩實名制，因此大多會在使用一次後進行拋棄，但由於許多國家沒有這個政策，因此我會建議你攜帶此工具，因為他能讓你的口罩不在放在口袋的順間失去效果。

An epidemic prevention gadget that even fewer people carry than the disinfection alcohol mentioned earlier, but I always bring it when I go out due to its convenience.

Since Taiwan has a mask rationing system mentioned many

times before, most masks will be discarded after using it once. However, because many countries do not have this policy, I would recommend that you bring this gadget because it can keep your mask from being put in your pocket and lost its effect instantaneously.

4. 額溫槍

Forehead thermometer

最少人會願意攜帶的設備，鑑於上述第二點臺灣在各大公司行號及觀光區域等位置在疫情期間皆有政策要求準備消毒酒精及額溫槍，故大多數臺灣人並不會攜帶，且由於使用此設備照射他人略顯無禮，故大多數人並不願意攜帶此用具，但如果你的國家除了醫院及公共場所外沒人在使用這項設備，那我建議你帶一下，他能增加你的保命機率。

This is an equipment with the least people willing to carry. In view of the second point above, Taiwan has the policy that in major companies and tourist areas disinfection alcohol and forehead thermometers are required in the premises, so most Taiwanese will not carry them. And because it is a bit rude to use this equipment on others, most people are unwilling to carry this equipment. Still, if no one in your country uses this equipment except in hospitals and public places, I will recommend you to carry it, it will increase your chance of survival.

最後我在這邊呼籲，如果說你並不是因為缺乏口罩而無法再外出時攜帶口罩，那我建議你還是**拋棄不戴口罩的舊有成見**，因為這個不起眼的東西能拯救你不被身邊不怕被感染的朋友傳染，那如果你沒有上述設備且**無法進行採購的話，那我建議你不要外出**，並參考下個章節的防疫技巧，他能幫助你安然度過瘟疫。

At last, I am here to call out. If you are not unable to carry a mask when you go out because of a lack of masks, then I suggest you abandon **the old stereotype of not wearing a mask**, because this inconspicuous thing can save you from the friends around you who are unafraid of being infected. If you do not have the above equipment and **cannot purchase it, then I would suggest you not to go out**, and refer to the epidemic prevention techniques in the next chapter, it can help you survive the virus safely.

防疫功夫

Disease Prevention Measures

如果你想防疫，你得要會這些招式

If you want to keep away from the virus, you should know this

新冠肺炎的傳播速度令人害怕，但它並非是無法防止被傳染的疾病，在這我將透過**過去臺灣的抗疫經驗及人們面對瘟疫時會做的保護動作**向你分享如何在此次瘟疫中生存的基本動作，動作如下：

The fast spread of coronavirus is terrifying, but it is not a disease that cannot be prevented from being transmitted. Here I will share with you how to deal with the virus through **the experience in fighting the epidemic in Taiwan and the protective actions** people will take when facing the virus. The basic actions for survival in the are as follows:

1. 用衣袖阻隔取代用手

Replace hands with sleeves

鑑於疫情未減，口罩成為人人必搶之物，只是若自己突然咳嗽或忍不住打噴嚏，身邊沒有口罩難免會引人側目，這時用衣袖阻擋噴嚏會是比用手阻擋是更優質的選擇，因為我們並不確定我們方才用手接觸的東西上是否有大量病毒，用衣袖阻擋會是更安全的選擇。此外，如果你可以接受用「Swag」姿勢阻絕噴嚏，那你還可以在防疫的過程增加一下你的時尚度，非常實用。

Because the epidemic situation has not decreased, masks have become a must for everyone. Still, if you suddenly cough or can't help sneezing, you will inevitably become the center of attention if you don't have a mask around. At this time, blocking the sneeze with your sleeve is better than blocking the sneezing with your hand, because we are not sure whether there are many viruses on the things we just touched with our hands. Blocking with sleeves would be a safer choice. If you can accept using the "Swag" posture to stop the sneeze, you can also increase your fashion level during the epidemic prevention process, which is very practical

2. 保持戰疫社交距離

Maintain social distance

雖說 2 公尺的社交距離並不能完全阻擋病毒（目前新研究的阻絕距離在 8 公尺），但它能減少你被傳染的可能，適當的與你的朋友保持有禮貌的社交距離，若他不能接受，那你也可以趁此向他宣導防疫意識，讓他知道你是因為重視他的安全而保持安全距離，不僅可以幫助自己，同時還能幫助他人。

Although a social distance of 2 meters does not entirely stop the virus (the current blocking distance in the new study is 8 meters), it can reduce the possibility of being infected. You should maintain a polite social distance with your friends. If he can't accept it, you can also seize the chance to promote the awareness of epidemic prevention to him, letting him know that you are keeping a safe distance because you value his safety. You can help not only yourself but also help others.

3. 用點頭或肢體語言取代接觸禮儀

Replace contact etiquette with nodding or body language

上個章節提到，新冠肺炎有接觸傳染的可能性，鑑於要有效防疫，在此我建議用肢體語言及點頭示意取代握手、親吻、擁抱的社交禮儀，這能幫助你與你的朋友不被外在可能的病毒傳染，是既有禮貌，又能關心別人的方式。此外，如果你是個漫威迷，你也可以考慮用「瓦甘達萬歲」的姿勢取代握手及擁抱，或者如果你是個科幻電影迷，你也可以考慮一下「瓦肯舉手禮」，雖然這個手勢有些難度，但他能降低你被接觸傳染的可能。

As mentioned in the previous chapter, COVID-19 has the possibility of transmission via contact. Given effective prevention, I would suggest using body language and nodding to replace the social etiquette of shaking hands, kissing, and hugging. This can help you and your friends not be infected by a possible external virus, which is a way of being polite and caring for others. In addition, if you are a Marvel fan, you can also consider using the "Waganda forever" gesture instead of handshake and hug, or if you are a science fiction movie fan, you can also consider "Vulcan Salute, "although this gesture is a bit difficult, it can reduce the possibility of you being infected through contact.

4. 到家記得消毒洗手

Remember to disinfect and wash your hands when you get home

這是防疫功夫中最關鍵的動作，在你不得不外出或與人社交完後，記得回家要為自己的手與衣服噴上酒精消毒，若是無法使用酒精，至少要完成用洗手乳或肥皂洗手的動作，這將是非常關鍵的消毒姿勢，他能降低你與你的家人被病毒感染的可能。

This is the most critical action in epidemic prevention. After you have to go out or socialize with others, remember to spray your hands and clothes with alcohol for disinfection when you go home. If you cannot use alcohol, you must at least use hand sanitizer or soap. The action of washing your hands is a critical disinfection action; it can reduce the possibility of you and your family being infected by the virus.

最後，若你認為上述動作在你的國家中有執行困難（國情與禮儀的不同容易導致防疫意識產生差異），那我建議你最少要**落實第四點且不要隨意外出**，因為就算你有落實上述的姿勢，但其他人不見得會遵守，當然！我還是建議你若**有機會能宣導就宣導，這能幫助你身邊的人**，也能幫助自己不被病毒侵襲。

Finally, if you think that the above actions are difficult to implement in your country (different national conditions and etiquette can easily lead to differences in awareness of epidemic prevention), then I will suggest that you at least **implement the fourth point and do not go out easily,** because even if you have applied the above gestures, but others may not have. Of course! I still recommend that **you promote the information if you have the opportunity.** It can help those around you and also help yourself not to be infected by the virus.

後記 Epilogue

臺灣是一個好地方嗎？

Is Taiwan a good place?

我覺得是！

I think so!

或許並不是所有人都了解臺灣，也或許並不是所有人都這麼認同臺灣，甚至大多數非臺灣人連臺灣跟泰國都沒有辦法分得清楚（臺灣英譯 Taiwan，泰國英譯 Thailand，因其發音相似，多數人在無字幕的情況下容易搞混，且國旗皆由紅、白、藍三大顏色組成，容易產生識別混淆），但這也是我想寫這本書的原因。

Perhaps not everyone knows Taiwan, and perhaps not everyone agrees with Taiwan so much. Most non-Taiwanese cannot even distinguish Taiwan from Thailand. (The English of Taiwan is Taiwan, sounding similar to Thailand in its pronunciation so that most people can confuse the two without subtitles, and the national flag of both countries are made up of the three colors of red, white, and blue, which is also prone to confusion), but this is why I want to write this book.

我想幫助臺灣被世界看見！

I want to help Taiwan to be seen by the world!

身為一個土生土長的臺灣人與一名連續創業者，我過去並非是一個太過「惜福」且「合群」的人，在許多看法上與決策上不僅與多數人有所不同，就連作法也大逕相庭，有時甚至還會大膽地跟身邊人批判國家政策與社會結構的問題，但鑒於臺灣是一個自由民主的國家，儘管我常常與身邊的朋友及合作夥伴抱持著不一樣的價值觀，但他們仍願意接受我的想法與我一同探討，甚至是會根據他們適合的狀況予以採納我的說詞。

As a native Taiwanese and an experienced entrepreneur, I was not a person who "cherishes the present" and "fit in a group" in the past. I differ from most people in many views and decisions and actions, and sometimes I even boldly criticize the problems of national policies and social structure with the people around me. With that being said, since Taiwan is a free and democratic country, even though I often hold different values with my friends and partners, they are still willing to accept my ideas and discuss them with me and even adopt my words when suited.

民主就是互相尊重及互相包容，這就是自由民主最高尚的價值，也是我身為臺灣人的驕傲。

Democracy is about mutual respect and tolerance. This is the noblest value of freedom and democracy. It is also my pride as a Taiwanese.

1971 年，中華人民共和國取得在聯合國的中國代表權，中華民國政府被迫退出聯合國以及包括世界衛生組織在內的聯合國下屬機構，失去與世界衛生組織相互間的官方聯繫。

In 1971, the People's Republic of China obtained the right to represent China in the United Nations. The government of the Republic of China was forced to withdraw from the United Nations and its affiliated agencies, including the World Health Organization, and lost official contact with the World Health Organization.

臺灣的主權及自由，在面對對岸泱泱大國的政治迫害下逐漸孤立無援，我們被迫離世界愈來愈疏遠，就連我們過去引以為傲的自由都隨時有可能面臨被摧毀的命運，過去臺灣遭異邦人統治的殖民陰影，將有可能在未來的某一日再次輪迴，臺灣，將有可能再次被吞噬。

Taiwan's sovereignty and freedom have gradually become isolated and helpless under the great power's political persecution on the other side. We are forced to become more and more alienated from the world. Even the freedom that we were so proud of may face the fate of being destroyed at any time. The shadow of being colonized and ruled by foreigners in the past may likely reincarnate again someday in the future, and Taiwan will likely be swallowed up again.

幸好！團結的人民與政府仍堅持不懈地為世界付出，不僅過去到現在會提供知識、技術給需要幫助的國家，更會在其他國家面臨自然災害時主動發起慈善援助，這些善良的人，讓臺灣得以發光，讓世界得以知曉。

Fortunately! United, the people and the government of Taiwan continue to work tirelessly for the world. They will provide knowledge and technology to the countries in need and take the initiative to provide charitable assistance when other countries are facing natural disasters. These kind people have made it possible for Taiwan to shine, and known to the world.

只要多一人知道我們的存在，那我們就多一分捍衛自由民主的希望。

As long as one more person knows our existence, then we have more hope in defending freedom and democracy.

在臺灣，我們有句話叫做：「臺灣最美好的風景就是人」。

In Taiwan, we have a saying: "The most beautiful scenery in Taiwan is people."

起初我不了解這句話的深刻含意，過去的我總認為這句話帶有嘲諷的意思，意指是只有臺灣人才會做出來的荒唐事件，而在我身上發生最嚴重的事件就是捲款事件了。

At first, I didn't understand the profound meaning of this sentence. In the past, I always thought this sentence was sarcasm, it meant the ridiculous incidents that only Taiwanese would do, and the most serious incident that happened to me was the abscond with money incident.

這是我過去在連續創業的歷程中，令我最難受的一次經驗，我遭到了多年夥伴的捲款，他的背叛與財產的流失讓我不得不中止我的創業計畫，這對當時的我來說無疑是非常大的一次衝擊，同時這也使我有非常長一段時間對臺灣人是抱持著厭惡且不願意再相信的態度（儘管我自己就是臺灣人）。

It was the most unpleasant experience in my past continual entrepreneurship experience. My work partner of many years absconded with my money. His betrayal and loss of property forced me to suspend my entrepreneurial plan. For me, it was undoubtedly a massive shock. At the same time, it also made me dislike Taiwanese and reluctant to believe others for a long time (even though I am a Taiwanese).

直到我第四次重新創業，當時我秉持著自己會撰寫計畫、架設網站與規劃設計的技能召集我過去的工作夥伴與老闆，但當時仍有服務技術及品質不足的問題。

Until I restarted my business for the fourth time, with the skills of writing plans, setting up websites, and planning and designing, I gathered my former work partners and bosses. However, there were still problems with insufficient service technology and quality.

在我躊躇不前時 Terry 出現了，他是丞信科技顧問管理有限公司的執行長，同時他也是一名專業的產業發展顧問，雖說當時他與我素昧平生，但他仍很願意透過他的專業及媒合解決我的困境，這讓我不僅能強化我服務的品質，更獲得更多有力的合作夥伴，大大強化了我創業的成功率。

While I was feeling hesitant, Terry showed up. He is the CEO of Chengxin Technology Consulting Management Co., Ltd., and he is also a professional industry development consultant. Although he and I had never met before, he was still willing to assist me in solving my predicament through his profession and matching service, which enabled me not only to strengthen the quality of my service but also obtained more powerful partners, which greatly enhanced my success rate in entrepreneurship.

再來就是被疫情影響的業務緊縮期間了，當時我正面臨網站缺乏轉換的問題時，Dean 及時出現了，他是我過去在平方夥伴行銷就職的老闆兼任我現在的行銷顧問，他不僅教授我搜尋引擎優化的技巧，更教授我操作網路廣告的技巧。終於，在他的悉心輔導下我獲得了第一張在疫情影響期間獲得的訂單，這不僅解決了我的生活困境，更讓我看到了持續經營的希望。

Then came the business contraction period caused by the epidemic. At that time, I was facing a lack of conversion on the website, and Dean appeared on time. He was my boss when I worked at Square Partner Marketing and my current marketing consultant. He not only taught me search engine optimization skills but the skills of operating online advertising. Finally, under his careful guidance, I got the first order I received during the epidemic. This not only solved my predicament but also gave me the hope of continuing business.

這時，令人備感巧妙的巧合出現了，正當我開始對持續創業這件事抱持著希望時，智庫雲端出版社的社長范世華出現了，他不僅邀請我一同製作這本書，更另外委託我與我的設計師 Tomy 一起為他設計他即將要出版的新書，這讓我非常的振奮，同時也讓我產生將臺灣人的友善分享給世界的想法。

At this time, an ingenious coincidence appeared. Just as I began to have hope again for continuing my entrepreneurship, Fan Shih hua, the president of the Think Tank Cloud Publishing House, appeared. He not only invited me to produce this book together, but also commissioned me along with my designer, Tomy, to design his upcoming new book for him, which makes me very excited, also given me the idea of sharing the friendliness of Taiwanese to the world.

「原來，臺灣最美好的風景真的是人。」

"It turns out that the most beautiful scenery in Taiwan is really the people."

最後我感謝我的摯友 Jerry Lin，感謝你一直以來聆聽我創業的想法與發展的計劃，這讓我更有動力堅持自己的道路，也感謝你在我缺乏靈感撰寫本書時告訴我不少我並不了解的知識與新聞動態，這不僅加速了我的著作時間，更賦予這本書臺灣人的靈魂。

Finally, I want to thank my best friend, Jerry Lin. Thank you for always listening to my entrepreneurial ideas and development plans. This makes me more motivated to stick to my own path. Thank you for telling me a lot of information and news updates when I lacked the inspiration during this book's writing process, which not only speeds up the time of my writing but also gifts this book the soul of Taiwanese people.

我是 Charles，臺灣是一個美麗、安全且充滿人情味的地方，我們歡迎你來。

I am Charles, Taiwan is a place that is both beautiful, safe, and full of hospitality, you are more than welcome to visit us!

國家圖書館出版品預行編目（CIP）資料

讓世界看見臺灣=Taiwan can help /莊博欽, 余慈雅作.
-- 初版. -- 臺北市 : 智庫雲端, 民109.10
面 ; 公分
中英對照
ISBN 978-986-97620-7-6(平裝)

1.傳染性疾病防制 2.病毒感染 3.臺灣

412.471 109014453

讓世界看見臺灣 Taiwan can help

作　　者　莊博欽 Charles Chuang、余慈雅 Julie Yu
出　　版　智庫雲端有限公司
發 行 人　范世華
封面設計　吳覺人
地　　址　台北市中山區長安東路 2 段 67 號 4 樓
統一編號　53348851
電　　話　02-25073316
傳　　真　02-25073736
E - mail　tttk591@gmail.com

總 經 銷　采舍國際有限公司
地　　址　新北市中和區中山路二段 366 巷 10 號 3 樓
電　　話　02-82458786 (代表號)
傳　　真　02-82458718
網　　址　http://www.silkbook.com

版　　次　2020 年（民 109）10 月初版一刷
定　　價　280 元
I S B N　978-986-97620-7-6